"In *The Cancer Generation*, John Geyman continues his provocative and disturbing full body scan of American health care by examining cancer care. Since 40% of us will be diagnosed with cancer in our lifetimes, the topic is not an abstraction and Geyman's report is not a pretty one. Commercialism, avarice and our painfully dysfunctional insurance system too often gang up to make a medical challenge a personal catastrophe. We can do better, he tells us once again."

—Fitzhugh Mullan, M.D.
Murdock Head Professor of Medicine and Health Policy, The George Washington University and Founding President of the National Coalition for Cancer Survivorship

"Having had considerable family experience with cancer and heart disease, and having just read John Geyman's *Do Not Resuscitate,* I had not expected to gain much from his new book, *The Cancer Generation*, but I was wrong. By concentrating here on the increasingly important issue of cancer in the United States, Geyman brings into sharp focus the problems of our multi-payer system in a way that not only clarified the issues in my mind but also bolstered my sense of urgency that we must establish a single-payer health care system. This book provides powerful ammunition toward that end because it presents with clarity much recently available factual information and valuable commentary on health care reform."

—Neil Davis, Ph.D.
Professor Emeritus of Geophysics, University of Alaska

"If you want an accurate diagnosis and practical treatment recommendations for a vexing and complex problem, you should seek the counsel of an experienced family physician who has carefully kept abreast of the latest scientific evidence. Dr. John Geyman here offers us his counsel on the vexing problems posed by America's broken health care system. While he focuses especially on cancer, most of his recommendations apply equally well to the other common chronic illnesses that afflict us."

—Howard Brody, M.D., Ph.D.
Director, Institute for the Medical Humanities,
University of Texas Medical Branch, Galveston, Texas

"No topic could serve as a better proxy for the deficiencies in the financing and delivery of health care in the United States than the ever increasing prevalence and expense of cancer. In *The Cancer Generation*, John Geyman describes the tragic and costly impact of the cancer burden, but then provides us with hope by describing a plan that would reduce these burdens of cancer."

—Don McCanne, M.D.
Past president, Physicians for a National Health Program
and PNHP Senior Health Policy Fellow

# THE WEATHER REPORT

## FORECAST:

## SEVERE STORM WARNING
Expect widespread damage and unnecessary deaths. A storm cellar won't protect you from cancer.

- Cancer soon to be nation's No. 1 cause of death

- Costs soaring out of control

- Decreasing access, increasing disparities

- Widening gaps in quality of care

- Insurance costs more and covers less

- Profit-driven market-based system is unaccountable and unsustainable

- Reform is blocked by powerful market stakeholders

- 79 million Baby Boomers face increased risk of cancer as they age, and will confront this challenge with dwindling resources

Projected Number of U.S. Cancer Cases
2000 Through 2050

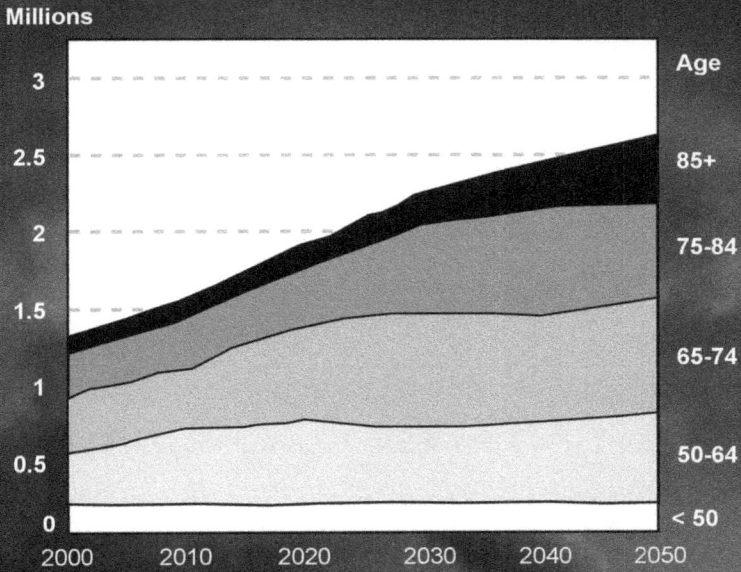

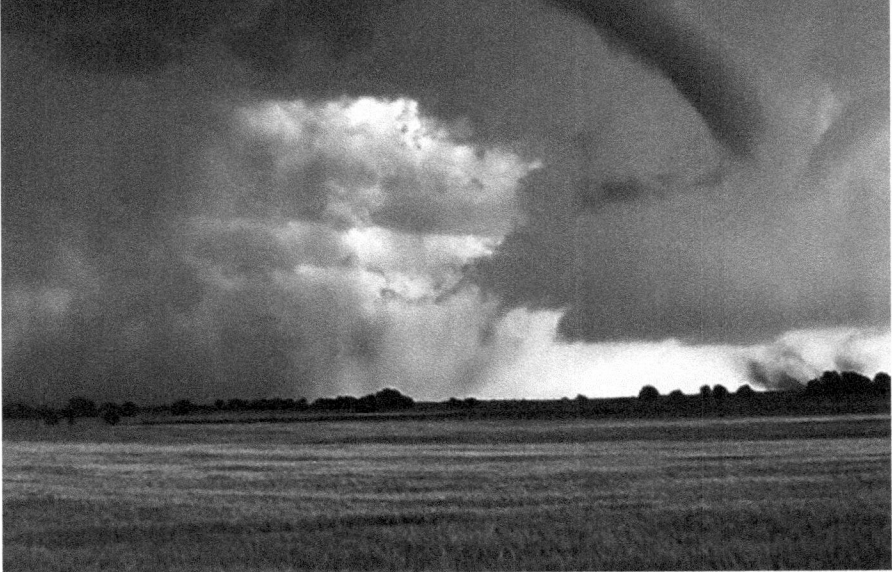

## Also By John Geyman, M.D.

*Family Practice: Foundation of Changing Health Care*

*Family Practice: An International Perspective in Developed Countries
(Co-Editor)*

*Evidence-Based Clinical Practice: Concepts and Approaches (Co-Editor)*

*Textbook of Rural Medicine (Co-Editor)*

*Health Care in America: Can Our Ailing System Be Healed?*

*The Corporate Transformation of Health Care:
Can the Public Interest Still Be Served?*

*Falling Through the Safety Net: Americans Without Health Insurance*

*Shredding the Social Contract: The Privatization of Medicare*

*The Corrosion of Medicine: Can the Profession Reclaim its Moral Legacy?*

*Do Not Resuscitate: Why the Health Insurance Industry is Dying,
and How We Must Replace It*

*Hijacked: The Road to Single Payer in the Aftermath of
Stolen Health Care Reform*

*Breaking Point: How the Primary Care Crisis
Endangers the Lives of Americans*

# THE CANCER GENERATION

## BABY BOOMERS FACING A PERFECT STORM

### Second Edition

John Geyman, M.D.

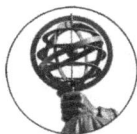

Copernicus Health Care
Friday Harbor, Washington

*The Cancer Generation: Baby Boomers Facing a Perfect Storm*

John Geyman, M.D.
Copernicus Healthcare
Friday Harbor, WA

Second Edition (CS)
Copyright ©2012 by John Geyman, M.D. All rights reserved

Book design, cover and illustrations by W. Bruce Conway
Cover photo by Mike Hollingshead
Author photo by Joseph (Bill) Reynolds, M.D.

Softcover: ISBN 978-1-938218-10-1
eBook: ISBN 978-0-9837734-2-9

Library of Congress Cataloging-in-Publication Data
is available from publisher on request.

Copernicus Healthcare
34 Oak Hill Drive
Friday Harbor, WA 98250

www.copernicus-healthcare.org
jgeyman@uw.edu

Printed by CreateSpace in the U.S.A.

## Dedication

For the millions of patients and their families dealing with cancer.

May we see the day when effective care is affordable and available to you based on medical need, and when all Americans have universal access to essential care without regard to income, race, or class.

# Contents

Tables and Figures ................................................................ 12

Acknowledgments ................................................................ 15

Preface      The Coming Storm: Will Care Be There for You? .......................... 17

## Part One: How Goes the War on Cancer?

Chapter 1      Cancer: How Big a Problem, and Are We Winning? ...................... 25

Chapter 2      New Technologies: A Balancing Act Between Benefits ................. 39
and Harms

Chapter 3      Cancer Care: Priceless, but Can We Afford It? ............................ 61

Chapter 4      Prerequisites for Availability of Effective Cancer Care ................... 81

Chapter 5      Lack of Access Harms and Kills ............................................. 99

Chapter 6      Do We Have the Best Cancer Care in the World? ...................... 113

Chapter 7      Major Challenges to Meet 21st Century Needs for ..................... 121
Cancer Care

## Part Two: How We Can Wage
## a More Effective War Against Cancer?

Chapter 8      In Sickness and in Wealth: How Distorted Markets ..................... 139
Build Wealth for the Few and Jeopardize Health for
the Many

Chapter 9      Financing Cancer Care: What Are the Options? .......................... 165

Chapter 10     Myths and Lies as Barriers to Health Care Reform ..................... 193

Chapter 11     A Way to Win: An Eight-Point Plan Based on National ............... 227
Health Insurance

Afterword      The Torch is in Your Hands: A Cross-Generational ................... 261
Message to Baby Boomers ............................................

Appendices

       1. Glossary ........................................................................ 263

       2. Selected Resources for Cancer Patients ............................... 277

       3. Frequently Asked Questions about Single-Payer National ........ 279
Health Insurance

       4. Advocacy Organizations for National Health Insurance ........... 283

Index ............................................................................................ 287

About the Author ........................................................................... 301

# Tables and Figures

Figure 1.1    Prevalence of Cancer by Age Group

Figure 1.2    Number of U.S. Cancer Cases, 2000-2050

Figure 1.3    Cancer Survivors in the United States, 1971-2002

Figure 2.1    Pathways by Which More Medical Care May Lead to Harm

Table 2.1     Costs and Benefits of Recently Approved Cancer Drugs

Figure 3.1    Underinsured and Uninsured Adults at High Risk of Going
              Without Needed Care and Financial Stress

Figure 3.2    The Average Income of the Top 5 Percent Has Doubled Since
              1980

Figure 3.3    Cumulative Changes in Health Insurance Premiums, Overall
              Inflation, and Workers' Earnings, 2000-2007

Figure 4.1    Top Cancer-Related Problems by Time Since Diagnosis

Table 4.1     Examples of Preference-Sensitive Cancer Decisions

Figure 5.1    Percentage of Office-Based Physicians Not Accepting New
              Patients According to Method of Payment, 2003-2004

Table 5.1     Cancer Screening by Health Insurance Status in Adults, 2005

Figure 5.2    Cancer Survival by Insurance Status

Figure 5.3    Consequences of Financial Costs of Cancer by Insurance
              Status

Table 7.1     General Guidelines for Cancer Screening Decisions in Older
              Adults

Figure 8.1    Health Insurance Oligopoly

Table 8.1     Investor-Owned Care: Comparative Examples versus Not-for-
              Profit Care

Table 9.1     Why Private Health Insurance Is Obsolete

Figure 9.1    How Much Would Uninsured be Willing to Pay for Coverage?

Table 9.2     Main Features of Single-Payer National Health Insurance

Figure 9.2    Health Costs as Percent of GDP: United States and Canada, 1960-2008

Figure 9.3    U.S. Public Spending Per Capita for Health is Greater than Total Spending in Other Nations

Table 9.3     What Americans Pay into the U.S. Health Care System Today

Table 9.4     Alternative Financing Systems and American Values

Table 10.1    Twelve Common Myths About U.S. Health Care

Figure 10.1   Annual Claims Distribution: The "20/80 Rule"

Table 10.2    Big 5 Health Insurance Industry Players, 2008

Figure 10.2   Big 5 Health Insurers: Share Performance, Week of February 23-27, 2009

Figure 10.3   Percentage Decline in Mortality from Amenable Causes and Other Causes from 1997-98 to 2002-03

Figure 10.4   Waiting Time to See Doctor When Sick or Need Medical Attention, Among Sicker Adults, 2007

Figure 10.5   Changes in Top Tax Rate in the U.S., 1918-2005

Table 11.1    An Eight-Point Plan for One-Tier Cancer Care

Table 11.2    Alternate Futures Based on Paradigm

Figure 11.1   Fundraising by U.S. Senators for the 2003-2008 Election Cycle

Figure 11.2   Administrative Costs: Single-Payer vs. Public Plan Option

# Acknowledgments

Through their support and encouragement, many colleagues have helped to make this book possible. I am especially indebted to these colleagues for their constructive comments and suggestions through their peer review of selected chapters:

- Don McCanne, M.D., past President of Physicians for a National Health Program and PNHP Senior Health Policy Fellow
- Frank Meyskens, M.D., Professor of Medicine, University of California Irvine and Director of the Chao Family Comprehensive Cancer Center
- Lee Newcomer, M.D., Head of Oncology Services at United Healthcare, Minneapolis, Minnesota
- Scott Ramsey, M.D., Professor of Medicine at the University of Washington and Full Member, Fred Hutchison Cancer Research Center, Seattle, Washington
- Roger Rosenblatt, M.D., Professor of Family Medicine, University of Washington
- John Saultz, M.D., Professor and Chairman, Department of Family Medicine, Oregon Health Sciences University, Portland, Oregon
- Joe Scherger, M.D., Professor of Family and Community Medicine, University of California, San Diego
- Stephen Taplin, M.D., Senior Scientist with the National Cancer Institute's Division of Cancer Control and Population Sciences, Applied Research Branch
- Richard Wender, M.D., past President of the American Cancer Society and Professor of Family and Community Medicine at the Thomas Jefferson University, Philadelphia, Pennsylvania

Many sources of reference materials were used in the course of research for this book. Reports from these organizations were especially helpful: the American Cancer Society, the Kaiser Family Foundation, the Commonwealth Fund, the Center for Studying Health System Change, the Pew Center for the People and the Press, the Center for Responsive Politics, the Medicare Payment Advisory Commission (MedPAC), the Centers for Medicare-Medicaid Services (CMS), the Medicare Rights Center, the Congressional Budget Office, the General Accounting Office, Physicians for a National Health Program (PNHP), and the World Health Organization (WHO). Thanks also to the publishers and journals who granted permission to reprint or adapt materials as cited throughout the book. I am especially grateful to Mike Hollingshead for his permission to use his graphic picture of an intense storm over Nebraska for the cover, which fits so well with the content of this book.

Virginia Gessner, my administrative assistant for more than 30 years, made major contributions to manuscript preparation. W. Bruce Conway, of Friday Harbor, Washington, was instrumental to this project from start to finish, including book design, cover and interior layout, preparation of all graphics, and typesetting of the 2009 and 2012 editions. Carolyn Acheson of Edmonds, Washington, did her usual excellent job with the index, and Andrew Seltser brought his practiced eye, carefully proofreading the entire manuscript. And as we brought out this updated second edition in 2012, Bruce Conway and Andrew Seltser were again instrumental to its conversion to Kindle ebook.

Finally, Greg Bates, as a skilled editor and publisher at Common Courage Press, helped me to better organize the book and make a complex subject more readable. His suggestions and encouragement have made this a better book than it would have otherwise been. And as always, my most thanks go to Gene, my wife, love and soul mate over these 56 years, who gracefully accepts my squirrel-away time in my study.

PREFACE

# The Coming Storm:
# Will Care Be There for You?

An explosion of romances after World War II gave birth to the baby boomer generation, and if we don't act now, cancer will be its closing chapter. On track to eclipse heart disease as the nation's number one killer, cancer as an issue will be front and center for this generation famous for changing the world.

The number one risk factor for cancer is aging: the older we get, the more likely cancer is to strike. In 2029, just 20 short years from now, the last of this generation will turn 65 and "baby boomer" will become synonymous with "senior citizen." Time for change is running short – for them and even shorter for their parents.

The dimensions of this crisis are already massive. Over a lifetime, 45 percent of men and 38 percent of women are expected to develop cancer, according to estimates by the American Cancer Society. Almost all of us know someone who has either died or survived cancer. More than 1.4 million Americans were newly diagnosed with cancer in 2008.[1]

As we will see, Baby Boomers face a fundamentally different disease from their parents and grandparents, one whose care has become big business driven by the need to satisfy investors to a degree never seen before in the disease's history. With the costs of cancer care rising much faster than other health care services, cancer care is becoming a financial vortex that is the medical equivalent of the subprime mortgage market. The 79 million-strong Baby Boomer generation will suffer a tidal wave of cancer and themselves pose a huge burden on society's health care budget. Between their growing numbers and the costs of their care, cancer will become the first major disease that, on its own, could overwhelm our health care system.

While cures for cancer dominate the headlines, signs abound that costs have grown so high that they threaten to eclipse concerns for care. In September 2007, the American Cancer Society (ACS) launched a public relations campaign that represented a radical shift from previous efforts. Where once it focused on smoking cessation and the importance of early screening for things like colorectal cancer, this campaign warned of a different menace: the impact of inadequate health insurance.[2] While not endorsing any particular health care reform plan, the ACS called for "4 As coverage" that can serve as our guide, our talisman, as we search for answers:

- *Adequate* –Timely access to the full range of evidence-based health care including prevention and early detection
- *Affordable* – Costs are based on the person's ability to pay
- *Available* – Coverage available regardless of health status or prior claims
- *Administratively simple* – Processes are easy to understand and navigate

The ACS further called for an end to cherry picking the health insurance market with the proposed recommendation that "a good health care reform plan must spread costs equitably among all those seeking insurance, whether they are healthy or not."[3]

A special report by the Kaiser Family Foundation and the American Cancer Society was released in February 2009 profiling the plights of 20 cancer patients less than 65 years of age who called in to the American Cancer Society's Health Insurance Assistance Service for help. This landmark report, *Spending to Survive: Cancer Patients Confront Holes in the Health Insurance System*, draws this conclusion:

"Even when people have private insurance, they may not be protected from high out-of-pocket costs if they are diagnosed with cancer. These costs, along with the cost of insurance premiums, can potentially force cancer patients to incur debt in order to pay for the care they need or forego or delay lifesaving treatment. Cancer patients who are unable to work due to their illness are particularly vulnerable, since they may lose their employer-sponsored insurance."[4]

But as good as this new urgency is, it doesn't quite encompass the nature of the beast we face. Five forces are now acting in concert: costs of cancer care are rising by more than 20 percent a year; there is an explosion of expensive new technologies of uncertain effectiveness; the quality of care in a profit-driven marketplace varies widely; political interference is preventing necessary reforms; and a wave of Baby Boomers with higher risks of cancer is starting to crest. As an oncologist and executive at UnitedHealthcare, Dr. Lee Newcomer looks at these trends and sees oncology being engulfed by a perfect storm.[5]

Many books expose the failings of our for-profit health care system. Yet few describe how this storm plays out for patients with cancer. We see the gathering clouds, embodied in familiar tragedies such as this story of Patricia, recounted by her father, Neil Davis, Ph.D. in his excellent recent book *Mired in the Health Care Morass: An Alaskan Takes On America's Dysfunctional Medical System for his Uninsured Daughter.*[6]

*At age 52, Patricia was a self-employed artist and part-time teacher living in Fairbanks, Alaska without health insurance. She had been insured most of her life by family policies during childhood and by her husband's employer-based policy as a university teacher. After a divorce and while struggling to make ends meet and raise her son, she went without health insurance for a time. As worries over being uninsured mounted, she took a part-time job with a small Alaska airline with the understanding that she would be eligible for health insurance after six months of employment.*

*Three months into the job, and after delaying a visit due to costs, she saw a physician with persistent symptoms and was diagnosed with cancer – small-cell lung cancer. Too close to the aorta, the cancer was inoperable. Her life turned upside down as she went into chemotherapy and radiation therapy. Medical bills approached $200,000 within a year, and the family was devastated by the disease and its costs. She was not eligible for Medicaid, and even after becoming totally disabled faced a two-year waiting period for Medicare. Despite her valiant efforts to combat the disease and the vigorous help of her family, she died after an 18-month course of treatment.*

All of this, including the lack of any safety net programs as her disease worsened and much more, make this book a compelling read. Variations of this story can be told by hundreds of thousands of Americans. Cancer is a scary diagnosis that makes us feel vulnerable and forces us to confront our own mortality. We hope to get effective treatment. Yet most of us know that even if we have health insurance, we can't assume that access to that treatment is available.

Regularly bombarded with news of spectacular breakthroughs in cancer screening, diagnosis and treatment, it might seem to some that we are on the road to winning the war against cancer. But with each passing year, the rising costs of care put the benefits of these advances farther beyond the reach of ordinary Americans.

Baby Boomers are becoming the generation in which better care reaches fewer people.

This book follows from my last book *Do Not Resuscitate: Why the Health Insurance Industry Is Dying, and How We Must Replace* It, which documents how necessary health care has become inaccessible for an ever larger part of the population. It also shows that our private health insurance industry goes to great lengths to avoid coverage of major illnesses such as cancer.

Other developments further raise the odds that lack of access to essential cancer care is getting much worse. Two examples suffice to illuminate the trends. It has become common for chemotherapy drugs to cost as much as $100,000 a year, often even more if combined with another drug. Second, there is now a new medical arms race heating up among U.S. hospitals over the purchase of proton accelerators. Each costs about $125 million, certain to drive up costs of treatment much higher, especially for prostate cancer, the second most common cancer among men.[7] These trends seriously compromise the ability of individuals, families, and even the health care system to afford essential cancer care. As the cost of drugs and the medical arms race for proton accelerators illustrate, we ration care on the basis of ability to pay, not by medical need. As Patricia and so many others have found, a safety net is often not available to help in dealing with this disease.

My previous books have dealt with our overall health care system,[8] its transformation by corporate interests,[9] the uninsured and our fragile safety net,[10] the privatization of Medicare,[11] the corrosion of medicine by business interests,[12] the failure and obsolescence of the private insurance industry,[13] how health care reform was hijacked by market forces in 2009-10[14], and the crisis in primary care.[15] This book examines the changing landscape of cancer in the U.S., including the extent to which the marketplace fails patients with cancer. We will ask whether the impacts of this market failure will force a paradigm shift in American health care, and if so, what directions that may take. In the last three chapters we will deal with some urgently needed directions for reform if we are to assure that all Americans who get cancer can receive effective care.

This second edition is done in order to update developments in the last two years since the first edition came out in print form. Areas of update particularly focus on increasing costs, decreasing affordability and access to necessary care, and further threats to the ability of patients with cancer to get essential care. We will also update the changing politics since the 2010 midterm elections as they relate to the current 2012 election cycle and the pressure building for needed reforms.

I have written about health care costs from several angles, always through the lens of a physician. Today I write with a different qualification, a different passion: I am a cancer survivor, just like many of you, just like your friends, like your parents and relatives, just like more than a third of all women and men will be over the course of their lives. I had metastatic testicular cancer at age 51, cured by surgery and the latest in chemotherapy. I feel the acute injustice of luck: why should I, or anyone else with such advantages, have access to all appropriate cancer treatment when so many others do not? Especially when the difference is a matter of life and death? When I say, I'm in this battle with you, I'm no longer talking just as a physician.

John P. Geyman, M.D.
January 2012

# References:

1.  Jemel A, Siegal R, Ward E, et al. Cancer Statistics, 2008. CA Cancer J Clin 58 (2): 71-96, 2008.
2.  Sack K. Cancer society focuses its ads on the uninsured. New York Times, August 31, 2007.

3.   American Cancer Society, Access to Health Care. We're taking action. Web site accessed June 21, 2008.

4.   Schwartz K, Claxton G, Martin K, Schmidt C. Spending to Survive: Cancer Patients Confront Holes in the Health Insurance System. Kaiser Family Foundation. Publication No. 7851, February, 2009.

5.   Newcomer LN. Oncology's perfect storm: The next decade. Amer J Managed Care 11 (17), Sup. S507-8, 2005.

6.   Davis N. Mired in the Health Care Morass: An Alaskan Takes On America's Dysfunctional Medical System for his Uninsured Daughter. Ester, AK, Ester Republic Press, 2007.

7.   Pollack A. Hospitals chase a nuclear tool to fight cancer. New York Times, December 26, 2007: A1.

8.   Geyman JP. Health Care in America: Can Our Ailing System Be Healed? Woburn, MA; Butterworth-Heinemann, 2002.

9.   Geyman JP. The Corporate Transformation of Health Care: Can the Public Interest Still Be Served? New York: Springer Publishing Company, 2004.

10.  Geyman JP. Falling Through the Safety Net: Americans Without Health Insurance, Monroe, ME: Common Courage Press, 2005.

11.  Geyman JP. Shredding the Social Contract: The Privatization of Medicare. Monroe, ME: Common Courage Press, 2006.

12.  Geyman JP. The Corrosion of Medicine: Can the Profession Reclaim Its Moral Legacy? Monroe, ME: Common Courage Press, 2007.

13.  Geyman JP. Do Not Resuscitate: Why the Health Insurance Industry is Dying, and How We Must Replace It. Monroe, ME, Common Courage Press, 2008.

14.  Geyman, JP. Hijacked: The Road to Single Payer in the Aftermath of Stolen Health Care Reform. Monroe, ME. Common Courage Press, 2010.

15.  Geyman, JP. Breaking Point: How the Primary Care Crisis Endangers the Lives of Americans. Friday Harbor, WA. Copernicus Healthcare, 2011.

# PART ONE

# How Goes the War on Cancer?

CHAPTER 1

# Cancer: How Big a Problem, and Are We Winning?

You can be sure that cancer will be part of your life. You'll either get it – nearly half of all men and more than a third of women will. Or you'll have a close friend who gets it, or be the child of someone who gets it, or the spouse of someone who has it, or in the worst-case scenario, be the parent of a child struggling with cancer. You cannot help but stand on the battlefield of the war against cancer. How America wages this war is leaving an indelible mark on your life.

Cancer is now on track to replace heart disease as America's leading cause of death within the next few years. This is a fight we have to win. Are we winning? And if we are off target, what changes are imperative for victory? Everything we discuss here focuses on these two questions.

Our views on how best to fight cancer are shaped by our efforts through history. Understanding the highlights of that struggle and its progress to date can widen our perspective on trends toward the future. This chapter therefore undertakes three goals: (1) to briefly touch on some historical landmarks in the cancer story; (2) to summarize cancer statistics today, together with what they can mean to real people; and (3) to consider conflicting views on how we're doing in the fight against cancer.

## Misperceptions Of Yesterday: Clues to Our Modern Blind Spots?

"You've got cancer." That dreaded phrase evokes fear, foreboding and anxiety. It is a disease that has exerted a special power on the human psyche for many centuries. From very early times in recorded human history, cancer has been the subject of great interest among people around the world. The first known written description of cancer is in an Egyptian papyrus from about 3000 B.C.[1]

Over the millennia to follow, in the absence of effective treatment, people have generated all kinds of theories and beliefs about its causation.

In the late 1700s in France, many people believed that cancer was a contagious disease spread by parasites. The first cancer hospital in the world was built in Reims, France, but it was forced to leave the city in 1779 because of the public's fear of contagion.[2]

Today, it is tempting to look back at that fear of contagion and see instantly the colossal distance we have advanced in our understanding since then. But in recalling some of what may appear as quaint foibles of a society struggling before the dawn of science, I want to pose a question to keep in the back of our minds: what views that we hold today might be seen in a similar light in the future?

The word "cancer" has interesting origins that are quite appropriate to what we have learned about the disease since it was first named. Hippocrates described non-ulcer forming tumors as "carcinos" and ulcer-forming tumors as "carcinoma." These words mean "crab" in Greek, suggesting an image of a crab's finger-like projections around itself. Carcinoma is the most common word applied to many cancers today.[3]

Against the long backdrop of human history, progress in real understanding and treatment of cancer is very brief – not much more than seven decades, with an increasing pace of developments since the 1970s. The benchmarks below share some characteristics. They all occurred within the last 75 years, they all mark big steps forward in a resolve to fight cancer, they all demonstrate just how recent our current efforts are, and they all hold out the promise of advance along with some actual advance. Yet despite these efforts our progress remains limited.[4]

- 1937 - President Franklin D Roosevelt signs legislation creating the National Cancer Institute (NCI) to support research related to the causes, diagnosis, and treatment of cancer.

- 1964 - The American Society of Clinical Oncology (ASCO) is established.
- 1971 - President Nixon signs the National Cancer Act of 1971.
- 1973 - For the first time, certification in medical oncology and gynecologic oncology is offered.
- 1989 - First offering of certification in radiation oncology.

- 1997 - The Cancer Genome Anatomy Project (CGAP) is launched, a multi-year project to assemble the first index of genes involved in cancer.

As one of eight federal agencies that together make up the Public Health Service in the Department of Health and Human Services (DHHS), the NCI's mission is to "reduce the worldwide burden of cancer through innovative research and development of ever better interventions to prevent and treat cancer." The National Cancer Act of 1971 broadened the scope and roles of the NCI to also include rehabilitation from cancer and the continuing care of cancer patients and their families. Since then, the NCI has coordinated the National Cancer Program.[5] The Act established 15 cancer centers for "clinical research, training, and demonstration of advanced diagnostic and treatment methods." There are now 61 such centers across the country.[6]

But returning to our question as to whether we have our own blind spots within this period of rapid technological advances, what could these be? Here are three obvious ones. Throughout this book, I will argue that we put too much faith in technology as the complete answer to cancer. We also overlook a crucial advance that, if implemented, could save lives right away: building a system of care that will deliver cancer care to all of us. Still another big blind spot: most of our interest and resources go to treatment, far more than to prevention of cancer.

## Cancer Today: The Gathering Storm Clouds

Despite waging an intense war against cancer since at least the 1970s, we could hardly have a bigger problem. As noted earlier, cancer has become the second leading cause of death in the U.S., and will replace heart disease as number one within just the next few years. Taken together, heart disease and cancer account for about one-half of all deaths in the country. Death rates from heart disease have been in sharp decline in the U.S. since 1950, even dropping by more than 6 percent between 2003 and 2004.[7] For Americans under the age of 85, cancer has already become the leading cause of death.[8]

As noted at the start of this chapter, the NCI estimates that almost one-half of men (45 percent) will get cancer over their lifetimes, together with 38 percent of women.[9] More than 1.4 million Americans were newly diagnosed with cancer in 2008, with more than half a million deaths from cancer in that year.[10]

Big as it already is, our cancer problem is growing. Since the incidence of cancer increases with age, the growth and aging of the population will lead to an increasing cancer burden, both for individual patients and their families, as well as for the health care system itself. The prevalence of cancer (newly occurring and existing cancers) among our population by age group is shown in Figure 1.1.[11]

FIGURE 1.1

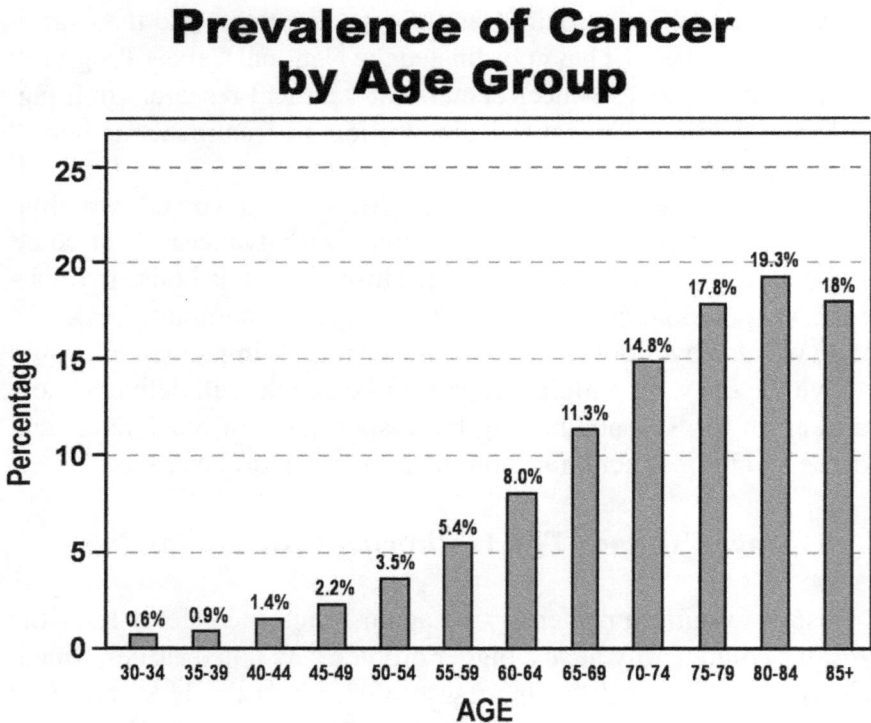

**Prevalence of Cancer by Age Group**

Source: Hewitt M, Greenfield S, Stovall E, eds. From *Cancer Patient to Cancer Survivor: Lost in Transition.* Washington, D.C. The National Academies Press, p 31,

The number of Americans 65 years of age and older has grown by almost 10 percent since 1995, is now 12.5 percent of the entire population, and is tracking toward becoming 20 percent by 2036.[12] Most new cancers and cancer deaths occur in people over 65.[13] The Institute of

Medicine projects that cancer cases will double from 2000 to 2050, especially for people over 75, as shown in Figure 1.2.[14]

## FIGURE 1.2

# Projected Number of U.S. Cancer Cases 2000 Through 2050

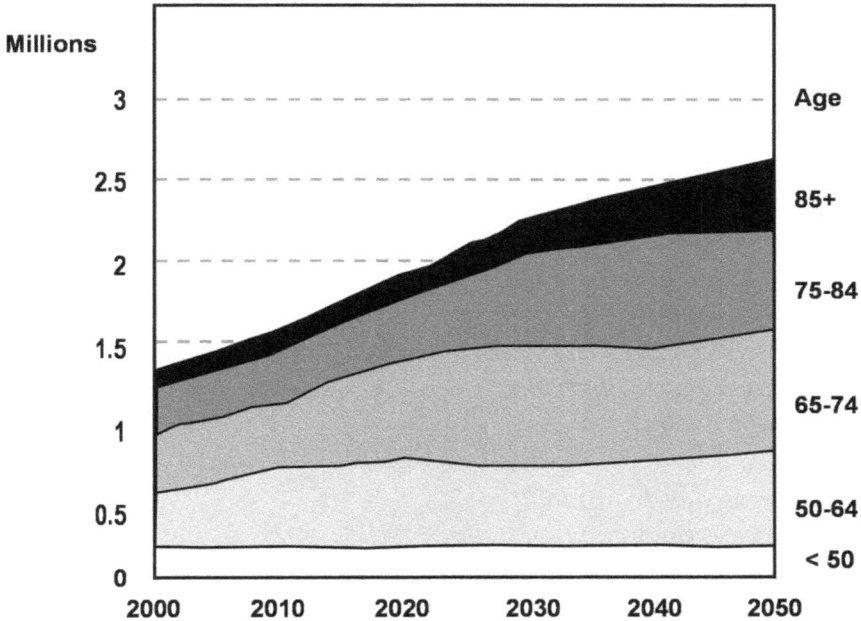

Source: Hewitt M, Greenfield S, Stovall E, eds. *From Cancer Patient to Cancer Survivor: Lost in Transition.* Washington, D.C. The National Academies Press, p 27,

The most common newly diagnosed cancers are prostate cancer for men and breast cancer in women. But lung/bronchus cancer is the number one killer for men over 40 and for women over 60. Breast cancer is the leading cause of death from cancer for women between 40 and 60. Just three cancers account for about one-half of all cancers among men – prostate, lung/bronchus, and colorectal; for women, the same except for breast instead of prostate.[15]

Cancer is not just pervasive, it's costly. The annual cost of cancer care is projected to increase by more than three-fold to $1,106 billion by 2023, more than for any other chronic disease. Cancer research is led and coordinated by the NCI, with an annual budget of almost $5 billion.[16] The 260 registered nonprofit organizations devoted to cancer outnumber all those devoted to heart disease, stroke, Alzheimer's disease, and AIDS put together. These charities raised more than $2.2 billion for cancer in 2005.[17]

All of the above are dry statistics that we can ignore but only at our peril. As Dr. Kerr White, well-known pioneer in health services, health statistics, epidemiology, public health, and medical education has observed: "Health insurance statistics represent people with the tears wiped off."[18]

Here is what cancer means to two of our fellow citizens, who appear in the February 2009 report by the Kaiser Family Foundation and American Cancer Society, Spending to Survive: Cancer Patients Confront Holes in the Health Insurance System.[19]*

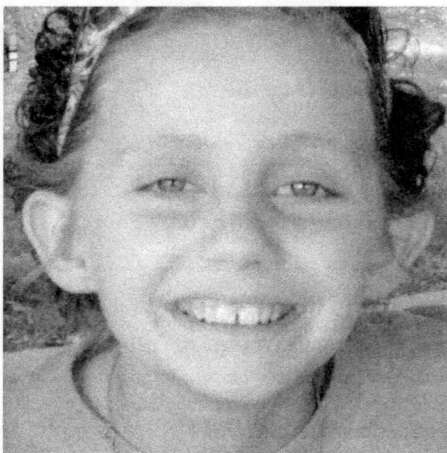

*Taylor Wilhite, age 10, was diagnosed in March 2007 with acute myeloid leukemia (AML), a fast-growing cancer of the blood and bone marrow. She received three rounds of chemotherapy and a bone marrow transplant; at one point she was taking 23 pills a day in addition to intravenous medications. Treatment has produced many side effects for Taylor – problems with her heart and hip, short-term memory problems, steroid-induced diabetes, and a compromised immune system. Taylor is insured through her father's job. She was approaching the $1 million lifetime maximum benefit for her insurance coverage. Her parents requested increasing the lifetime maximum, and the insurer agreed to increase the maximum to $1.5 million. However, Taylor's doctors have said that even this higher maximum will not be sufficient to cover her additional surgeries. Taylor's parents are tracking*

*her medical expenses because the insurance company does not provide notification of the total spent until after the lifetime limit has been reached. Although Taylor is in remission, she will need follow-up visits with her oncologist every two months, checkups with her endocrinologist every three months, and multiple major surgeries on her hip.*

* Patient stories and picture reprinted with permission from the Henry J. Kaiser Family Foundation. The Kaiser Family Foundation is a non-profit private operating foundation, based in Menlo Park, California, dedicated to producing and communicating the best possible information, research and analysis on health issues.

"The insurance has been good, we just never expected Taylor to reach the lifetime maximum on her benefits," says Taylor's mother, Amy. "It has been a lot of work to keep up with the medical expenses and figure out what to do next."In addition to treatment costs, the Wilhites have been burdened by travel costs. During the four months that Taylor was in Cincinnati for her bone marrow transplant, her father drove 10 hours roundtrip each weekend to visit her. Once she reaches her plan's maximum, Taylor will become HIPAA-eligible. HIPAA coverage will cost more than her current insurance and will present a financial burden to the family of six; they have started reducing their household expenses by discontinuing nonessential utilities such as cable and Internet.

...

*Michael Courtney, 41, was diagnosed with cutaneous T-cell lymphoma, a rare form of non-Hodgkin lymphoma, in 2007. The cancer had started on his tongue and quickly spread. Michael received radiation and chemotherapy. His treatment will continue indefinitely.*

*Michael is an auto mechanic, and had been hesitant to switch employers for fear that he would not be able to continue his treatment without health insurance coverage. But he eventually made the change when his new employer offered him immediate benefits. He elected the same insurance company that he had at his previous job. His new insurance plan is offered through Healthy New York, a state-supported program aimed at expanding lower-cost private coverage among individuals and small employers.*

*One month after switching employers, Michael learned that his new policy excluded his pre-existing condition. The insurer was able to consider the cancer a pre-existing condition because Michael did not have 12 months of continuous coverage prior to changing jobs. A full year of continuous coverage is required under the federal HIPAA rules that govern pre-existing condition exclusions for employees who switch to a new employer. Michael was continuously insured for nine months with his previous employer. The insurer denied any claims that were made after Michael switched jobs, and he found himself strapped with unanticipated medical debt. Michael was paying for coverage, but could not get the treatment he needed.*

*Michael's girlfriend, Maddie, called the insurer to find out what happened. 'I was crying and trying to get them to understand what we were going through, but they didn't care,' Maddie says. "We didn't want to lie down and not do anything. Michael's life was on the line."*

*Michael could get an individual, guaranteed issue policy, but he would face a three month waiting period for his pre-existing condition. Meanwhile, the premium to elect COBRA was more than he could afford. Michael decided to delay his treatment for three months until he exhausted his pre-existing exclusion period.*

## Are We Winning the War on Cancer?

First, some good news. There is no question that cancer, in most of our lifetimes, has gone from an incurable disease – a virtual death sentence – to a point where many cancers can be cured, and for those not cured, a chronic disease for survivors.

The most dramatic improvements in outcomes have been in children. For children with cancer, the odds of survival were less than 25 percent in the 1960s. Today that figure has jumped to about 80 percent, with some types of cancer in the mid to high 90 percent range.[20]

The incidence rate for cancer has declined since the early 1990s.[21] Moreover, overall death rates for all cancers have shown modest reductions over the last 30 years. Despite the growth and aging of our population, the number of cancer deaths actually declined for two years in a row from 2005 to 2007.[22] And another remarkable change is the steady increase in the number of cancer survivors as indicated by Figure 1.3.[23] There are now more than 10 million Americans who are cancer survivors, about 3.5 percent of the population.

The probability of long-term survival depends on many factors,

FIGURE 1.3

## Cancer Survivors in the United States 1971 - 2002

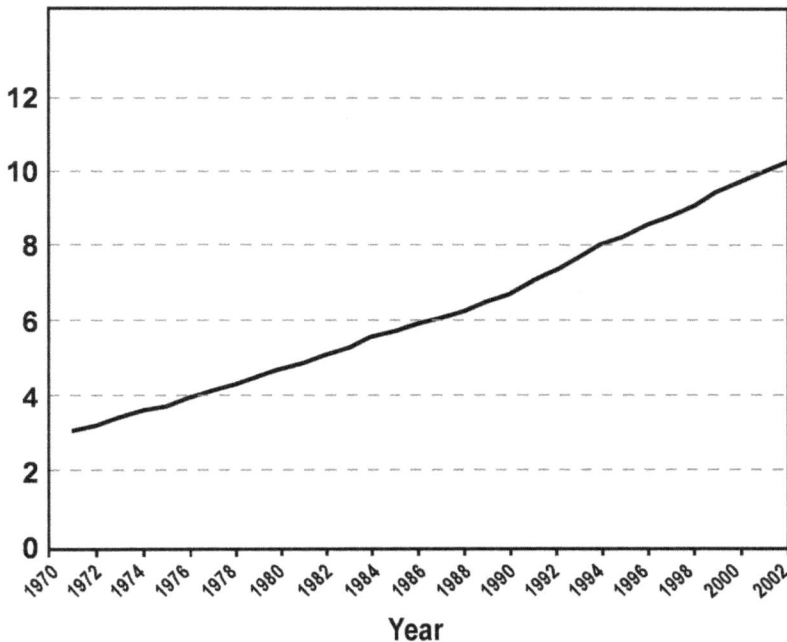

**Year**

Source: Hewitt M, Greenfield S, Stovall E, eds. From *Cancer Patient to Cancer Survivor: Lost in Transition.* Washington, D.C. The National Academies Press, p 25,

including age, cancer type and stage, and whether or not one has other illnesses, or co-morbidities. Once cancer patients have survived for one year, their odds of surviving another five years rise. Once past that first year mark, they are more likely to survive for five years than is someone newly diagnosed with cancer.[24]

In its 2008 *Annual Report to the Nation on the Status of Cancer* (issued jointly with the National Cancer Institute, the Centers for Disease Control and Prevention, and the North American Association of Central Cancer Registries), the American Cancer Society reported that the rate of cancers being diagnosed in the U.S. between 1999 and 2005 dropped by 0.8 percent each year for both men and women combined. In addition, the death rate from cancer declined by 1.8 percent a year between 2002 and 2005, almost twice the 1.1 percent decrease seen from 1993 through 2002. Although death rates for some cancers increased (esophagus and bladder among men, pancreas among women, and liver among both men and women), cancer death rates decreased for 10 of the 15 most common cancers among both men and women.[25]

Moreover, the Dallas-based National Center for Policy Analysis (NCPA), drawing from a 2007 article in *Lancet Oncology*,[26] reports that U.S. cancer care is Number One in the world. To achieve this ranking, cross-national five-year survival rates for the period 2000 to 2002 were measured. Among the findings:[27]

- For all cancers, American women have a 63 percent chance of living at least five years after a cancer diagnosis, compared to 56 percent of European women; for American men, 66 percent can expect to live at least five years after diagnosis, compared to 47 percent for European men.

- Compared to Canada, for all cancers between 2001 and 2003, five-year survival rates for American women were 61 percent compared to 58 percent for their Canadian counterparts; the same comparisons for American men were 57 percent versus 53 percent in Canada.

All of this sounds as if we are well on our way to winning the war against cancer in this country. Betsy McCaughey, an economist with the NCPA, drew this conclusion from this study:

"International comparisons establish that the most important factors in cancer survival are early diagnosis, time to treatment and access to the most effective drugs. Some uninsured cancer patients in the United States encounter problems with timely treatment and access, but a far larger proportion of cancer patients in Europe face these troubles. No country on the globe does as good a job overall as the United States. Thus, the U.S. government should focus on ensuring that all cancer patients receive timely care rather than radically overhauling the current system."[28]

Although the above still sounds as if we are doing very well in our battle against cancer in this country, there are growing concerns in the opposite direction. In its 2008 *Cancer Trends Progress Report*, the NCI has listed these important ways, among others, in which the nation is losing ground in the fight against cancer:[29]

• Incidence rates of cancer of the liver, pancreas, kidney, esophagus, and thyroid have continued to rise, as have the rates of new cases of non-Hodgkin lymphoma, leukemia, myeloma, and childhood cancers. Incidence rates of other cancers are also increasing (e.g., brain, bladder, melanoma in women, and testicular).

• Lung cancer death rates in women continue to rise, though not as rapidly as before. Death rates for cancer of the esophagus and thyroid in men as well as of the liver are also increasing.

• Unexplained cancer-related health disparities remain among population subgroups. As one example, African-Americans and people with low socioeconomic status have the highest rates of both new cancers and cancer deaths. In fact, a 2008 study of more than 13,000 patients with breast, prostate, and colorectal cancer found that lower socioeconomic status is a risk factor for more advanced disease and higher mortality for all three cancers.[30]

The claim by some that the U.S. has the best cancer care in the world does not seem credible when we look at how far short we fall in making effective care available to all Americans with cancer. Recognizing this, the NCI established the Center to Reduce Cancer Health Disparities in 2001. And in 2007, the American Cancer Society launched its 4 A's program to promote universal access to cancer care, mentioned earlier, that is *adequate, affordable, available,* and *administratively simple.*[31]

For now, what can we make of these conflicting views about the quality of our cancer care? While it may be tempting to conclude from the *Lancet Oncology* report mentioned above that our cancer care is second to none, that study's dependence on five-year survival rates does not tell the whole story. Health service researchers tell us that a cross-national study to answer that question would have to control, at a minimum, for age, sex, and stage of cancer in each country, which was not done in that study. Although we can probably conclude that we do more cancer screening than is done in many other countries, that study does not clarify who is number one in terms of lower cancer mortality and quality of life along the way. Both are more reliable outcome measures than five-year survival rates, which are inherently subject to various kinds of bias. In Chapter 6 we will describe how survival rates are biased and examine in some detail how cancer care in this country stacks up compared to other advanced countries around the world.

Meanwhile, we can only expect that the disparities within our population will only get worse as our economic downturn deepens, and as cancer care becomes less affordable and accessible to those in need, and what little safety net we have unwinds further. As this is written, for example, a decision has just been made to close outpatient oncology services at the University Medical Center in Las Vegas, Nevada and cut out Medicaid coverage for chemotherapy drugs.[32]

## Closing Comment

From becoming the leading cause of death to becoming a growing problem among an aging population, cancer is one of our biggest challenges. Many pin their hopes on a straightforward solution. Technology is widely seen as THE silver bullet in this war against cancer. Can it win the war, and if so, at what cost? We will address those questions in the next chapter.

# References:

1. Some key events in the history of cancer. Emory University Winship Cancer Institute Web site. www.cancerquest.org/index.cfm?page=2405, accessed July 3, 2008.
2. ACS. The history of cancer. ACS Web site htpp://www.cancer.org/docroot/CRI/contentCR, accessed July 3, 2008.
3. Ibid # 2
4. NCI. The National Cancer Institute: More than 70 years of excellence in cancer research. NCI Web site http://www.cancer.gov/aboutNCI/excellenceinresearch, accessed July 3, 2008.
5. NCI. NCI mission statement. NCI Web site http://www.cancer.gov/aboutncimissionstatement, accessed July 3, 2008.
6. Vanchieri C. National Cancer Act: A look back and forward. *J Natl Cancer Inst* 99 (5): 342, 2007.
7. STATbite. Major causes of death in the U.S., News. *J Natl Cancer Inst* 99 (3): 194, 2007.
8. Jemel A, Siegel R, Ward, E, et al. Cancer Statistics, 2008. CA *Cancer J Clin* 58 (2): 71-96, 2008.
9. Ibid # 8.
10. Ibid # 8.
11. Hewitt M, Greenfield S, Stovall E, eds. *From Cancer Patient to Cancer Survivor: Lost in Transition.* Washington, D.C. The National Academies Press, p 31, 2006.
12. Ibid # 8.
13. Ibid # 6.
14. Ibid # 11, p 27.
15. Ibid # 8.
16. Bodenheimer T, Chen E, Bennett HD. Confronting the growing burden of chronic disease: Can the U.S. health care workforce do the job? *Health Affairs* 28 (1): 65, 2009.
17. National Center for Charitable Statistics: A program for the Center of Nonprofits and Philanthropy at the Urban Institute. Washington, D.C., National Center for Charitable Statistics, 2006.
18. White KL. Health care research: old wine in new bottles. *Pharos Omega Alpha Honor Med Soc*, 56: 12-16, 1993.
19. Schwartz K, Claxton G, Martin M, Schmidt C. *Spending to Survive: Cancer Patients Confront Holes in the Health Insurance System.* Kaiser Family Foundation and American Cancer Society, KFF Publication No. 7851, February, 2009.
20. McGregor LM, Metzger ML, Sanders R, et al. Pediatric cancer in the new millennium: Dramatic progress, new challenges. *Oncology* 21 (7): 809-20, 2007.
21. National Cancer Institute. *Cancer Trends Progress Report – 2007 Update.* Report Highlights. U.S. National Institutes of Health. Washington, DC: 2008.
22. Ibid # 6.
23. Ibid # 11, p 25.

24. Ibid # 11, p 61.
25. ACS News Center. Cancer death rates and incidence down, annual report shows. Atlanta, GA. American Cancer Society, November 25, 2008.
26. Verdecchia A, Fransiso S, Brenner H, et al. Recent cancer survival in Europe: a 2000-02 period analysis of EUROCARE-4 data. *Lancet Oncology* 8: 784-96, 2007.
27. McCaughey B. U.S. cancer care is number one. Brief Analysis No. 596. Dallas, TX. National Center for Policy Analysis, October 11, 2007.
28. Ibid # 27.
29. Ibid # 21.
30. Byers TE, Wolf HJ, Bauer KR, et al. The impact of socioeconomic status on survival after cancer in the United States. American Cancer Society, on-line June 25, 2008.
31. American Cancer Society, Access to Health Care. We're taking action. Web site accessed June 21, 2008.
32. Wells A. Added Medicaid cuts raise concerns. UMC loss might hit $20 million. *Las Vegas Review-Journal*, November 22, 2008.

## CHAPTER 2

# New Technologies: A Balancing Act Between Benefits and Harms

"I fear, from the experience of the last twenty-five years, that morals do not of necessity advance hand in hand with the sciences."[1]

—Thomas Jefferson, 1815

New technologies in cancer care have helped to lengthen the lives of many people with cancer, and even led to cures for some. Curative treatment is now possible for a number of cancers, including testicular cancer and Hodgkin's disease. Other newer technologies are not curative, but can extend survival with good quality of life as a chronic disease, as illustrated by this patient's experience.[2]

*Tom, 65, was diagnosed with a rare leukemia, and was told that he might live another three years. He was treated with imatinib (Gleevec), one of the new "targeted therapies" which gained FDA approval in 2001. Gleevec was designed to silence growth signals inside cancer cells, turning cancer into a chronic disease. Three years later, Tom was able to return to work as a truck driver, at a cost of $3,100 a month for Gleevec. Fortunately, he had coverage under Medicare, and has been doing well seven years after diagnosis of his leukemia.*

Our faith in medical technology is fully justified by examples such as this one. But for all the triumphs of modern cancer care, there are also many examples of marginal outcomes, or even harms, as a result of increasingly expensive and unaffordable care. Some of our newer technologies are not as effective as we are led to believe. Do we have an accurate assessment of the value of new technologies in our fight against cancer? We can't make judgments about how important technologies are based on anecdotal success stories. We need an accurate assessment of the value of new technologies in our fight against cancer.

This chapter raises four questions: (1) how do new technologies influence medical care?; (2) how do we separate and assess their benefits and harmful impacts?; (3) how much value are we getting from these new technologies?; and (4) are we in denial about the limitations of technology for curing cancer? These four questions form the heart of our focus here.

## Medical Technologies:
## How Do They Influence Medical Care?

Cutting edge technology may be all about the "new new thing," but the taxonomy for how we can best think about it was laid out brilliantly over 35 years ago. Lewis Thomas (1913-1993) was a renaissance man in American life. Over his remarkable career in medicine, including serving as Dean of two medical schools (Yale and New York University) and as President of the Memorial-Sloan Kettering Institute, he was also highly respected as a poet, etymologist, and essayist. He is perhaps best known for his collection of essays *The Lives of the Cell: Notes of a Biology Watcher*, in which he described these three levels of technology:[3]

- *Non-technology* – non-curative care for patients with advanced diseases (e.g., intractable cancer, advanced cirrhosis)
- *Halfway technology* – also care that is non-curative but may delay death (e.g., liver or heart transplants)
- *High technology* – curative treatment or effective prevention techniques (e.g., polio vaccination)

By his discerning classification, most of our new medical technologies are not in the high category, but instead fall into the halfway and non-curative technology arenas. These are important nonetheless when they succeed in adding time, especially if it is quality time, to a patient's life.

New technologies may at times be cost-effective if they replace more costly interventions, as occurred during the late 1970s when CT scanning on an outpatient basis avoided some hospital admissions for patients with suspected brain tumors.[4,5] But more often than not, new technologies, independent of their effectiveness, are additive to other interventions and increase the volume and cost of medical care.

Because of the high stakes involved, patients facing the prospects of cancer are especially vulnerable to accepting treatment at whatever the risks or costs. In this stressful situation, the need for excellent judgment and informed decision-making about the potential benefits and risks of alternative treatment approaches could not be more important. In their landmark article in 1999, Drs. Elliott Fisher and Gilbert Welch, from their base at the Center for the Evaluative Clinical Sciences at Dartmouth Medical School, described the many ways in which more medical care can be harmful. Figure 2.1 shows their conceptual framework of pathways, whether through more diagnosis or more treatment, that can lead to worry, disability, unnecessary

FIGURE 2.1

# Pathways by Which More Medical Care May Lead to Harm

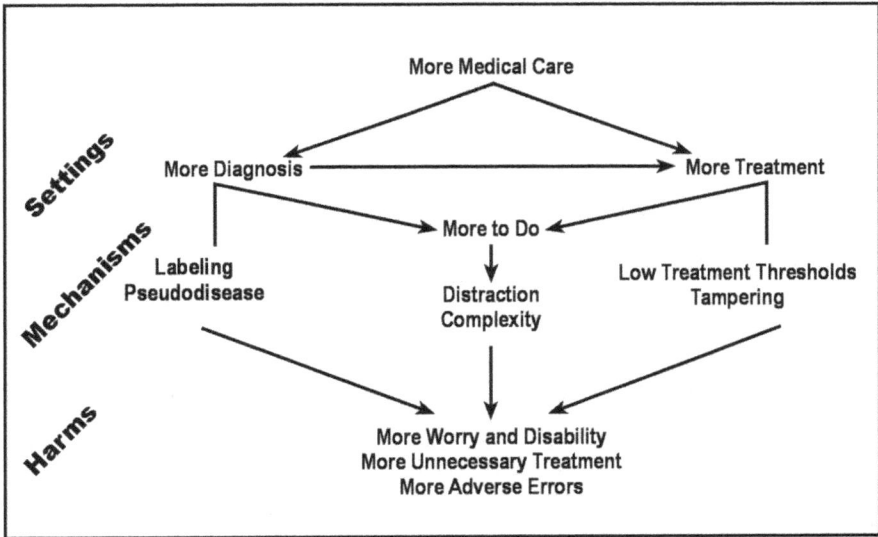

Source: Reprinted with permission from Fisher ES, Welch HG. Avoiding the unintended consequences of growth in medical care: How might more be worse? *JAMA* 281 (5): 446-53, 1999.

treatment, medical errors, and adverse events.[6]

We will see many examples in this book where more medical care results from early diffusion into the marketplace of new technologies for screening, diagnosis, and treatment of cancer. Some of this care is useful, and some is not. As diagnostic tests become more sensitive, for example, they often give false-positives, leading to a cascade effect of more testing and even inappropriate, unnecessary, or harmful treatment.

## New Technologies In Cancer Care:
## Benefits Versus Harms

The pace of new technologies being added to the armamentarium of cancer care grows more rapid all the time. There are about 400 new cancer drugs in the pipeline at the moment (many with a price tag of about $50,000 a year), robotic surgery is being used for some cancers, genetic testing is being marketed for screening purposes, and a brand new area of research and development – nanotechnology (involving molecular-sized particles) – holds promise to take currently available methods of diagnosis and treatment to a whole new level, both in terms of effectiveness and expense. And, despite widespread belief that the FDA is a tough regulator that slows approval and demands that drugs must be cost effective, these new technologies are being brought to market quickly, in keeping with our American way, with virtually no regard for demonstrated cost-effectiveness. We will return to this discussion in later chapters. Table 2.1 lists some examples of cancer drugs recently approved by the FDA.[7]

Despite the many success stories of modern cancer care, there are many other examples of marginal outcomes, and even harms, from the application of new technologies. Before we can make a one horse bet on technology, we need to look at its failures and drawbacks as well as its successes. This quick tour of some of the recent technological developments in screening, diagnosis, and treatment of cancer illustrate some of the pros and cons of these advances.

### Diagnostic and Prognostic Tests
### *Genetic Testing*

The last 15 years have seen a flurry of activity in identifying genes associated with various cancers. As examples, BRCA 1 was the first gene associated with breast cancer to be cloned. It has been found that HER2, a gene on the surface of breast cancer cells, can be effectively targeted by trastuzumab (Herceptin), a monoclonal antibody approved

## TABLE 2.1

# Costs and Benefits of Recently Approved Cancer Drugs

| Recently Approved Cancer Drugs | Approximate Cost of I Month of Treatment ($)* | Median Overall Survival Benefit in Randomized Clinical Trials (Months)† | Other Benefit† |
|---|---|---|---|
| Advanced non-small cell lung cancer progression after platinum-based chemotherapy Erlotinib | 3,200 | 2 | |
| Advanced colorectal cancer Bevacizumab Cetuximab | 5,500 10,000 | 4.7 Not Established | |
| Myelodysplastic Syndrome Lenalidomide Azacitidine | 7,000 6,000 | Not Established Not Established | Reduced Transfusion Dependence |
| Metatastic renal cell carcinoma Sunitinib | 4,000 | Not Established | |

\* Source: for costs: Medical Letter or Drugstore.com
† Physician's Data Query, National Cancer Institute
Source: Ramsey SD. How should we pay the piper when he's calling the tune? On the long-term affordability of cancer care in the United States. J Clin Oncology 25 (2): 176 , 2007.

by the FDA in 1998 for the treatment of metastatic breast cancer. In women with advanced breast cancer, HER2 is overproduced in at least one in four of them. Because of these findings, diagnostic tests are being used to identify those women who have over-expressed HER2 and will respond to Herceptin.

While in many instances the HER2 test can better tailor chemotherapy for the individual patient, there are several problems. Herceptin is expensive. If it's going to be used, it had better be needed. But quality control is lacking in many laboratories, so that tests may not be valid. In fact, the quality control is so poor that several studies have found false-positive and false-negative results, each in the sizeable range of about 20 percent. This translates into the likelihood that a test is accurate little more than 50:50. Current evidence-based clinical guidelines restrict the use of Herceptin to patients testing positive for the HER2 gene. Yet many oncologists don't use the test, putting patients on Herceptin who are unlikely to respond to treatment, exposing them to needless risk and expense.[8] UnitedHealthcare, for example, has found that while only 4 percent of its enrollees' oncologists haven't been using the test, an additional 8 percent were inappropriately treating *under*-expressed patients.[9]

In addition to helping cancer drugs (especially biologics) to be targeted to individual cancer patients, genetic testing is now being promoted for widespread screening for various cancers. Although only a minority of cancers are believed to be hereditary (eg., about 10 percent for breast cancer), mutations in the genes BRCA1 and BRCA2 are known to increase the risk of women getting breast cancer from a lifetime risk of about 13 percent to about 50 to 85 percent. These same genes also increase the odds of ovarian cancer from less than a 2 percent lifetime risk to 20 to 50 percent.[10]

While gene mutations can be identified, at least experimentally, for a growing number of other cancers, including colorectal, prostate, gastric, and melanoma, they do not yet provide clinically useful results that can change treatment. There is still a lack of clinical research to know how best to use many of the results of genetic testing.

The use of genetic testing for screening purposes carries unavoidable risks and harms. If such tests reveal a mutated gene which increase one's risk of cancer down the road, the patient then has to deal with a new level of fear and anxiety about the future. Such results are also nearly certain to lead to further procedures and testing, much of it unnecessary. Here is an all too frequent sequence: First, BRCA1 and BRCA2 are detected. Since they are known to increase the risk of cancer in the opposite breast and of ovarian cancer, they lead many oncologists to recommend more frequent mammography and perhaps

MRI screening, together with transvaginal ultrasounds and CA-125 blood tests every six months to detect ovarian cancer. This seems inherently logical: test more when the risks rise. There's just one catch: the increased testing has no impact on survival.[11]

Here's one example that shows why this apparently ironclad logic fails. The Laboratory Corporation of America began marketing a new screening test for ovarian cancer, OvaSure, under development at Yale University, before its clinical utility had been validated. The Society of Gynecologic Oncologists raised concerns about its accuracy and warned that some women may end up having their ovaries removed unnecessarily. In October 2008, the FDA also became concerned, asked the company to cease marketing, and will require FDA approval before it can be marketed further.[12]

Screening for prostate cancer is even more complicated. A 2008 report of a study by researchers at Wake Forest University of more than 4,000 Swedish men found five variants of genes in men with prostate cancer, each raising a man's lifetime risk of getting that cancer by 10 to 20 percent. If a man has a family history of prostate cancer, as well as all five variants, his risk for prostate cancer goes up by about 10-fold.[13] How should we act on this information? The answer seems obvious: jump on it and treat preemptively. Yet this is another fascinating case of infallible logic actually being fallible.

Prostate cancer has two unusual features: most are slow-growing, and most men get it if they live long enough, as autopsy findings confirm. Although some prostate cancers are aggressive and rapidly growing, the likelihood of their occurrence cannot be forecast by genetic testing. Despite this, a new test is soon to be released, through Wake Forest University, to conduct genetic testing by analyzing DNA in blood and saliva, at a cost of less than $300. Even though it won't detect the likelihood of an aggressive prostate cancer, this test is likely to be very popular. We can anticipate that many men will become needlessly anxious from the results, leading to more diagnostic procedures, and unnecessary potentially harmful treatment. Dr. Peter Albertson, a prostate cancer specialist at the University of Connecticut, calls this "the boutique medicine of the future," adding that "there is already too much prostate cancer screening resulting in too much treatment. We are just feeding off of this cancer phobia."[14]

Although still lacking demonstrated clinical utility, genetic testing is surging ahead as a business venture. A shift is taking place in thinking about cancer treatment – toward using genetic information to "personalize" chemotherapy to the genetic makeup of the individual patient, and away from the "one size fits all" approach. Drug manufacturers are pursuing this line of research, not just to help identify patients who will respond to their drugs, but also in hopes of salvaging older drugs which were not previously successful.[15] But there is a downside to this marketing hype, as Ellen Matloff, director of genetic counseling of the Yale Cancer Center, points out:

"The negative fallout includes an alarming increase in patients who did not receive appropriate informed consent before having testing, and whose tests were interpreted incorrectly by their well-meaning health care providers. Misread tests could lead women to undergo unneeded surgery."[16]

### CT Scanning
Computerized tomography (CT) has revolutionized diagnostic radiology over the past 30 years. At least 62 million CT scans are performed every year in the U.S., including at least 4 million in children, up by more than 20-fold since 1980. About one-half of scans in adults are of the full-body for screening purposes.[17]

Other CT scans in common use are for colorectal cancer (virtual colonoscopy) and for early detection of lung cancer in adult smokers. Virtual colonoscopy (also known as CTC or CT colonography) costs between $500 and $1,500, less than a standard colonoscopy. If polyps are found, a standard colonoscopy is still required in order to remove them.[18] In view of its limitations, CTC is not covered by either Medicare or many private insurers as a cancer screening procedure. In February 2009, CMS announced that "there is insufficient evidence to conclude that CTC improves outcomes for Medicare beneficiaries."[19]

None of these CT scans has received approval by the FDA or the American College of Radiology for screening purposes. Clinical evidence for the benefits of these procedures is still lacking, but their use continues to grow each year. Imaging centers have become the latest "cash cow" in the medical industrial complex, and many are owned by the physicians prescribing their use. Full-body CT screening procedures are promoted for asymptomatic adults at a cost of about $800 to $1,500 for each scan.[20]

The profligate use of these scans without evidence of clinical benefit not only wastes money, they carry health risks. A 2007 report by leading radiation physicists called attention to the risks of radiation exposure, especially of full-body CT scans. They estimate that current CT usage may account for as many as two percent of all cancers in this country.[21] In addition, CT scanning inevitably leads to a cascade of follow-up tests and procedures as the "fishing trip" continues on in the quest to find more clinical problems which are not yet symptomatic.

### *Ultrasound and MRI Breast Cancer Screening*

While mammography has been an important step forward in screening for breast cancer, it does miss some cancers. As a result, ongoing efforts to refine the accuracy of screening has led to the use of ultrasound and/or MRI to improve the yield of screening. Ultrasound is less expensive (about $100) and less sensitive. MRI is more expensive (about $1,000) and more sensitive. Both methods find more cancers, but there are questions as to how they best fit into screening for breast cancer.

Two recent large studies give some indication of how much these methods add to the diagnosis of breast cancer. A study of 969 women with cancer in one breast and normal breast examination and mammogram of the other breast found that MRI screening found an additional 30 biopsy-proven cancers in the opposite breast (3.1 percent).[22] In another study of 2,637 women, mammography alone found 7.6 cancers per 1,000 women screened, while mammography plus ultrasound found 11.8 cancers per 1,000 women screened.[23]

Both methods, however, have many false positives, cause patients further anxiety, and may lead to unnecessary biopsies. In an effort to clarify the role of MRI screening for breast cancer, the American Cancer Society issued guidelines in 2007 recommending that only women at high risk (lifetime risk of cancer of 20 percent or higher) should have an annual MRI as well as an annual mammogram.[24] These guidelines specified these high-risk factors, including women with a known BRCA mutation, women who are untested but have a first-degree relative with a BRCA mutation, and women who were treated with radiation to the chest between 10 and 30 years of age.[25]

## Cancer Therapies
### *Targeted Therapies*

Medical treatment for cancer has for decades involved intravenous chemotherapy intended to kill rapidly dividing cancer cells but unfortunately also kills cells in some normal tissues. Although still the treatment of choice for many cancers, traditional cytotoxic chemotherapy is starting to give way to a new generation of targeted therapies, which are now a component of treatments for many cancers, including lung, breast, colorectal, pancreatic, lymphoma, leukemia, and multiple myeloma.[26] The promise is simple yet alluring: kill the cancer cells, preserve the health patients have, and improve survival rates.

There are two kinds of targeted therapies – monoclonal antibodies (eg., Avastin) and small molecular inhibitors (eg., Gleevec). They can allow treatment to be individually tailored to patients with specific molecular targets, hopefully to kill cancer cells and spare normal cells.[27]

Targeted therapies have become one of the latest advances in cancer treatment, generating high excitement throughout the cancer care community. Of the new anticancer drugs approved by the FDA since 2000, 15 have been targeted therapies while only 5 have been traditional chemotherapy drugs.[28] Targeted therapies have come into widespread use quickly, well before their efficacy and value have been established by clinical research. When added to traditional chemotherapy in multi-drug regimens, costs climb exponentially, often with marginal benefits to patients. But do patients get a good bang for the buck out of these expensive treatments? This experience, as described by Dr. Lee Newcomer, oncologist at UnitedHealthcare, the nation's second largest insurer, illustrates some of the problems with targeted therapies, both for the individual patient and the system itself.

"Last year I became aware of a UnitedHealthcare patient with breast cancer who was being treated in private practice with both Avastin and Herceptin. By the end of the year, her treatment bills totaled $160,000. There was no proof whatsoever that those two drugs work together. There's only a theoretical possibility. This patient's oncologist – a private practitioner – decided to try the combination. The patient was employed in a small firm – six employees. Under small-group insurance law with guaranteed coverage, her employer's health insurance rates increased dramatically. The company could not afford the increase, and it was unable to find any other carrier with affordable rates because of its claim history for this patient. As a result, the employer dropped coverage, and all six people who worked for that company are now uninsured. I use this story to illustrate the fact that when a doctor starts to experiment with their hugely expensive new drugs, the ramifications go far beyond that one individual patient."[29]

Many cancer drugs are used for indications beyond FDA approval – so called "off-label" use. Why is that a problem? Several reasons: they are usually very expensive (up to $10,000 a month), they may not be safe or effective, and they typically have toxic side effects. But off-label use is widespread practice. The drug industry welcomes broader use of its products, and as we will discuss in later chapters, prescribing physicians also have financial conflicts-of-interest encouraging off-label use. The Bush Administration maintained a permissive regulatory environment allowing off-label cancer therapies to flourish in the name of innovation. In fact, the rules under which Medicare decides reimbursement policies were further relaxed in the waning weeks of the outgoing Administration. Under heavy lobbying pressure from industry and some professional groups, new Medicare rules were adopted in November 2008 that expand the number of drug compendia, or reference guides, used to determine Medicare coverage from one to four. Some of these guides have close financial ties to the drug industry. Medicare now requires only one of these guides to recommend coverage, thereby expanding off-label coverage even without clinical evidence of effectiveness.[30]

### *Anti-Anemia Drugs*
The 1990s hailed an important breakthrough in a new class of drugs called Erythropoesis-stimulating agents (ESAs). These address anemia, a common problem among cancer patients when they are undergoing chemotherapy. Developed by Amgen, they increase the number of red blood cells and help to reduce the need for blood transfusions. They

have been widely marketed for use in cancer patients for the last seven years or so. But the safety of the three major drugs in this group, Epogen, Aranesp and Procrit, has recently been called into question.

It now appears that ESAs carry serious risks themselves. The drugs have seen widespread use, potentially putting much of the cancer patient population at risk. A 2008 report by Dr. Charles Bennett at Northwestern University Feinberg School of Medicine, together with colleagues around the country, evaluated 51 clinical trials over a ten-year period. It found that patients receiving these drugs had a 57 percent higher risk of having venous thromboembolism (blood clots). More importantly, patients had a 10 percent higher mortality rate compared to patients not receiving ESAs.[31] The mechanisms involved in these risks are not yet clear, and further research is underway. In July 2008, the FDA ordered re-labeling of these drugs to say that they should not be used for cancer patients receiving chemotherapy when a cure is anticipated, or when hemoglobin levels are 10 grams per deciliter or higher.[32]

### Proton Therapy

In the same way that targeted therapies have the potential to revolutionize chemotherapy, proton therapy holds the same potential to revolutionize radiation therapy for cancer. Instead of using x-rays as in traditional radiation therapy, proton beams are accelerated by a cyclotron to about two-thirds the speed of light and targeted more precisely on cancer tissue than on surrounding normal tissues. Proponents claim that radiation exposure is reduced compared to x-ray therapy and that normal tissues are spared more effectively with this technique.[33]

But there are drawbacks suggesting that tighter regulation and further study are needed. Like targeted therapies, proton therapy is spreading like wildfire across the country in advance of solid evidence that they it will meaningfully extend the lives of patients being treated. It holds another characteristic in common with targeted therapy: they're both extremely expensive. Proton accelerators weigh in at 222 tons, and are housed in buildings the size of a football field with walls up to 18 feet thick. They have been called "the world's most expensive and complex medical device." Each costs upward of about $125 million. Their cyclotrons use magnetic fields to accelerate protons, which are then focused by electromagnets on a 21,000-pound magnet that rotates

360 degrees around the patient to position a nozzle that directs the proton beam to the cancer.[34]

There is a new medical arms race heating up among hospitals and even private medical practices as they jump to adopt this new technology. There was only one proton center in the country until 2000 (at Loma Linda Medical Center in California). Today there are five, more than a dozen are being planned (including two in Oklahoma City and two in Chicago suburbs). Still others are being considered as vendors and investment firms aggressively promote these centers. ProCure Treatment Center is a leading company involved in promotion, financing, building, and operation of these facilities. ProCure's first project is being built in Oklahoma City for two medical practices with a total of six oncologists.[35]

While proton therapy is being proposed by its supporters for the treatment of many cancers, especially those of the head and neck, eye and orbit, and cancers in children, there is a potentially huge and lucrative market fueling rapid construction of these centers: prostate cancer. The numbers tell the story: Medicare pays about $50,000 for proton therapy for prostate cancer, nearly twice what it pays for x-ray radiation therapy.

Despite this rapid diffusion of proton therapy into the medical marketplace, however, an economic analysis by the Fox Chase Cancer Center in Philadelphia projects that proton therapy will be cost-effective for only a small subset of prostate cancer patients. Critics argue that proton centers, as a lucrative new profit center, will be over-utilized for the wrong reasons, and will greatly increase the cost of cancer care. Dr. Anthony Zeitman, radiation oncologist at Harvard and Massachusetts General Hospital (which has its own proton center), worries that this development is "the dark side of medicine."[36]

### Nanotechnology

Even as the cancer care industry has yet to establish roles of new technologies based on cost-effectiveness and demonstrated improvements in outcomes for patients, the newest development – nanotechnology – will carry these challenges of implementing promising technologies with little regard to effectiveness or cost to yet another level. Many types of nanoparticles are under development which can be conjugated with several functional molecules simultaneously, such as tumor-specific ligands (i.e., a signal triggering molecule binding to a site on a target protein), antibodies, anticancer drugs, and imaging probes. They can be used for specific delivery of anticancer agents, detection of circulating cancer cells, and monitoring of treatment results in real time. Nanoparticles are 100 to 1,000-fold smaller than cancer cells.

Multifunctional nanoparticles may push cancer treatment closer to individualized therapy, detecting malignant cells, pinpointing and visualizing their location by real-time imaging, and killing the cancer cells with minimal toxic side effects.[37] Some nanoparticles do not depend on drugs at all, but instead destroy cancer cells by physical means. As one example, gold nanoshells either absorb or scatter light. The shells are built on a silica core, upon which a very thin layer of gold is painted. After trillions of these nanoshells are injected into the patient's bloodstream, they can be targeted by a blast of infra-red, thereby heating up the particles and killing tumor cells. This process, called photothermal ablation, is in early clinical trials in Texas by Nanospectra Biosciences.[38] When these kinds of new technologies come into general use, we can only expect the costs of cancer care, if they follow the trends discussed above, to jump exponentially. Whether they are worth that cost will depend on their effectiveness, which won't be known for years to come.

It would be easy, but wrong, to characterize the cautions raised on these technologies as an argument against the role of advancing technology in curing cancer. The role it can play, while constantly oversold by businesses seeking to profit from it, is still vital to our winning the war on cancer. The above examples, however, show that technology development requires sufficient regulation and quality control to maximize its benefits and minimize its harms.

## Value In Cancer Care: How Much Do We Need?

Debate over value – of what we get for our money in cancer care – has only barely begun in this country. Real debate is long overdue, and we still haven't even decided on benchmarks or criteria of value. Are we to measure progress in our war against cancer by how much money is raised and spent on this effort? By survival of those who can afford care? By how we compare with other industrialized countries by outcomes of care? By quality-adjusted life years (QALYs) that account for quality as well as length of life? Are we deploying our resources for the benefit of individual patients or our entire population?

These questions go mostly unanswered as a polarized debate continues over cancer policy without any consensus over measures of success. In our deregulated marketplace, industry stakeholders have long had the upper hand in bringing new products to market, often without much research confirming their efficacy and safety. We have earlier seen examples of the anti-anemia drugs and proton therapy centers. Industry consistently advocates for continuation of today's pattern of marketing and early adoption of technologies, regardless of their costs. Industry stakeholders fight for "off label" use of their products and fight against application of any measures of cost-effectiveness. Obligated to investors and urged on by Wall Street analysts, they closely guard their prerogatives to set prices as high as they can.

Dr. Thomas Roberts was formerly a practicing oncologist at the Massachusetts General Hospital before leaving practice to become a hedge fund manager for Noonday Global Management in Charlotte, North Carolina. Here is how he sees our present political landscape:[39]

"We currently find ourselves in an environment where the innovative pharmaceutical and biotechnology companies that discover and develop new so-called targeted therapies for cancer and other serious diseases have the power to charge what the market will bear, particularly in the United States. At least for now, that means that they can charge very large sums for these new products.

There are two consequences of the current situation. First, because profit margins can be very high for successful products, companies doing work in cancer have been able to attract a tremendous amount of investment capital. Cancer drugs now in the pipeline now outnumber the next two most-represented therapeutic classes combined. The second consequence is that expenditures on cancer drugs are growing rapidly. A study by Cohen and Company, a Wall Street investment firm, estimates that growth rates for targeted cancer drugs will be almost 20 percent per year – among the highest in all of medicine."[40]

Concerning the cost of Avastin, typically about $100,000 a year for chemotherapy, Sally Pipes, an economist and president of the San Francisco-based conservative think tank, the Pacific Research Institute, argues that we get high value regardless of the cost:

> "There's an old story about a frog who lives at the bottom of the well. One day, he looks up and sees a tiny circle of sky above him. 'Ah,' he says to himself, 'now I've seen the world.' The argument that drug prices are driving up health care costs is as disconnected from reality as that frog at the bottom of the well. ...In reality, prescription drugs reduce medical spending... by obviating the need for prolonged hospital stays, surgery, and other expensive procedures like anesthesia. It's time to climb out of the well and cast some sunlight on this pervasive myth." [41]

Despite this claim of value, however, the use of Avastin in lung or breast cancer does not obviate the need for other treatments and does not significantly prolong survival.[42]

Practical examples occur every day in cancer care of the increasing tension between market stakeholders, payers and patients as buyers of their products. As an example, how are we to decide about use of a Taxol/Avastin regimen that adds two months of life for $160,000 a year, especially when the quality of life is poor because of drug toxicity?[43]

Faced with spiraling costs of cancer care as we are, other industrialized countries are grappling with the cost-effectiveness challenge and tackling the issue head-on. In England, for example, the National Institute for Health and Clinical Excellence (NICE) takes cost-effectiveness into account in setting policy from a societal perspective. Sir Michael Rawlins, chairman of NICE, has this advice for us on this matter:[44]

> "The United States will one day have to take cost effectiveness into account. There is no doubt about it at all. You cannot keep on increasing your health care costs at the rate you are for so poor return. You are 29th in the world in life expectancy. You pay twice as much for health care as anyone else on God's earth."

Whether public or private, payers need to be sure that benefits of products and services justify their payments.

Oncologists are caught in the middle, finding themselves in a marketplace culture where "anything at all costs" prevails. A recent national survey found that four of five oncologists believe that costs should not enter into treatment decisions for individual patients, and they seem to accept QALYs in the range of $300,000 a year, at least six times higher than most experts think is reasonable and affordable.[45] By way of comparison, cardiac bypass surgery has been well accepted as a clinically beneficial procedure with a QALY of $25,000 to $30,000. While it is still unknown what we can afford as a system for general medical care, as well as for cancer care, there will be real limits in the not too distant future.

Practicing oncologists are in a double-bind – first, by being reluctant to be the "bad guy" by denying patients the option of treatment when it is unlikely to be effective, or even futile; and second, by often having financial conflicts-of-interest (COIs) acting as incentives for providing these treatments. Current reimbursement policies give them incentives to offer more cycles of treatment and avoid painful discussions with patients about stopping treatment. It has been common practice by manufacturers of chemotherapy and anti-anemia drugs to give large rebates to prescribing oncologists based on the volume of drugs purchased and whether they use one company's products exclusively. To be fair, the high cost of these drugs requires oncologists to make sound business decisions about the volume of drugs to be purchased if they are to have a financially viable practice, but the current policies of drug manufacturers places oncologists in a conflict-of-interest situation. These rebates can make a big difference in their practice income. For example, one oncology practice in the Pacific Northwest, with six oncologists, received $1.8 million in rebates in one year, all over and above reimbursement from Medicare or private insurers for administering the drugs.[46]

A growing number of oncologists are concerned about the spiraling costs of cancer care, decreasing access to care, the unsustainability of these trends, and how their own practices are beset with conflicts of interest about their roles as treating physicians. Arthur Caplan, a bioethics professor at the University of Pennsylvania, calls this "one of the toughest issues in oncology, since drug prices can involve 'exchanging family assets' for the possibility of a few more months of life."[47]

# How We (Don't) Set Policy:
# A Dance Of Denial About Limits

As we have seen, the market is setting cancer policy by default. As a society, we have not been able to come to grips with the tradeoffs necessary to make affordable and effective cancer care available to all Americans. Most of our resources are going into treatment, much of which is yielding only marginal outcomes, while the prevention side is being underemphasized and under-funded. We do make explicit trade -offs in other areas of health care based on cost-effectiveness, such as for cardiac bypass surgery mentioned earlier. We tend to question the use of treatments with QALYs over $50,000. But cancer continues to be "special". Payers are reluctant to deal with a "cancer taboo", which makes it difficult for them to deny payment for treatments, even when they are of limited or no benefit.

So a dance of denial about limits goes on. We can hardly expect cancer policy to be set by individual patients and their physicians. We should, however, be able to expect responsible government to do so. But we have not yet given the Center for Medicare and Medicaid Services (CMS) the authority to use cost-effectiveness as an essential criterion for coverage and reimbursement policies, and as we will see in a later chapter, the FDA is in large part beholden through user fees to industry that it is supposed to be regulating. Meanwhile industry and cancer advocacy groups lobby politicians and government for their own special interests.

These efforts have at times been carried to extremes. Death threats sent to physicians provide one striking example of this extreme. These doctors were targeted because they advised the FDA not to approve a new drug, Provenge, for use against prostate cancer. Presumably the threats came from patients with prostate cancer wanting access to the drug. But the doctors' reasoning was solid: while a small study had suggested Provenge might increase survival of men with advanced prostate cancer, evidence was too limited to warrant its approval.[48]

The downside of letting cancer policy continue to be set by market forces escalates all the time. Access and outcomes can only get worse as prices of care continue to surge. The advent of genetic medicine further raises the stakes of policy running adrift. As Dr. James Evans, medical geneticist at the University of North Carolina, observes:

"Today, medical science is at another such threshold with the advent of individualized medicine. Driven by advances in genomics, emerging insight into each individual's unique susceptibility to disease promises to transform patient care. However, such advances will also compel a fundamental restructuring of the way medical care is delivered in the United States... the emergence of individualized medicine, driven primarily by advances in the ability to dissect the individual's genome, undermines this traditional system. By learning to identify an individual's risks, the individual becomes less attractive to insure for the very maladies for which they require coverage... the solution is for all to pool their risks."[49]

As an oncologist and insurance executive, Newcomer has these suggestions for more explicit and sustainable cancer policy:[50]

"Policy needs to address several questions. One, how cost-effective must the gain in life be? Two, how much is the ceiling for pricing a drug without competition? Three, how do we control and learn the most from off-label usage? We have to make trade-off decisions. We do not have unlimited resources."

Important as new technologies are to care of cancer, we are starting to see that each new advance further stresses our delivery system in complex and interrelated ways. Increased cost limits access and affordability, raising questions about the value of care, how to ensure equitable access to care, and how payers (whether patients and their families or private and public insurers) can finance that care. We will return to these questions in later chapters. But for now, we turn to the next chapter to better understand how many people are being left out of our market-based system for cancer care.

# References:

1.  Thomas Jefferson to M Correa de Sierra, 1815, Memorial Edition 14: 331.
2.  Szabo L. Cost of cancer drugs crushes all but hope. *USA Today* July 10, 2006.
3.  Thomas L. *The Lives of a Cell: Notes of a Biology Watcher*. New York: Bantam Books, 1975.
4.  Larson EB, Omenn GS. The impact of computed tomography on the care of patients with suspected brain tumor. *Med Care* 5 (7): 543 – 51, 1977.
5.  Larson EB, Omenn GS, Loop JW. Computed tomography in patients with cerebrovascular disease: Impact of a new technology on patient care. *Am J Roentgenol* 131 (1): 35-40, 1978.
6.  Fisher ES, Welch HG. Avoiding the unintended consequences of growth in medical care: How might more be worse? *JAMA* 281 (5): 446-53, 1999.
7.  Ramsey SD. How should we pay the piper when he's calling the tune? On the long-term affordability of cancer care in the United States. *J Clin Oncology* 25 (2): 176 , 2007.
8.  Culliton BJ. Interview: Insurers and 'targeted biologics' for cancer: A conversation with Lee N. Newcomer. *Health Affairs Web Exclusive* 27 (1): W-41-W-51, 2008.
9.  Personal communication, Dr. Lee Newcomer, March 6, 2009.
10. Hobson K. Tracing cancer connections: Genetic testing for yourself and family members can both create and alleviate fear. *HEAL* 2 (2): 35-42, Summer 2008.
11. Ibid # 10.
12. Pollack A. FDA says cancer test failed to get its approval. *New York Times,* October 9, 2008: B3.
13. Zheng L, Sun J, Wiklund F, et al. Cumulative association of five genetic variants from prostate cancer. *N Engl J Med* 358: 910-19, 2008.
14. Kolata G. $300 to learn risk of cancer of the prostate. *New York Times*, January 17, 2008: A1.
15. Winslow R, Chase M. Genetic research may help pick patients' best cancer drugs. *Wall Street Journal*, June 2, 2008: B4.
16. Chase M. Cancer-gene test boosts Myriad's sales. *Wall Street Journal*, May 7, 2008: B5.
17. What's NEXT? Nationwide Evaluation of x-ray Trends: 2000 computed tomography. (CRCPD publication no. NEXT_2000CT-T) Conference on Radiation Control Program Directors, Department of Health and Human Services, 2006.
18. Rundle RL. CT scans gain favor as option for colonoscopy. *Wall Street Journal,* October 28, 2008: D1.
19. Pollack A. Medicare blow to virtual colonoscopies. *New York Times*, February 13, 2009: A18.
20. Pennachio DL. Full-body scans – or scams? *Medical Economics*, August 9, 2002: 62-71.
21. Brenner DJ, Hall EJ. Computed tomography – An increasing source of radiation exposure. *N Engl J Med* 357: 2277-84, 2007.
22. Lehman CD, Gatsonis C, Kuyh CK, et al. MRI evaluation of the contralateral

breast in women with recently diagnosed breast cancer. *N Engl J Med* 356: 1295-1303, 2007.

23. Berg WA, Blume JD, Cormack JB, et al. Combined screening with ultrasound and mammography vs mammography alone in women at elevated risk of breast cancer. *JAMA* 299 (18): 2151-63, 2008.

24. Matthews AW. When a mammogram isn't enough. *Wall Street Journal,* June 24, 2008: D1.

25. Saslow D, Boetes C, Burke W, et al. American Cancer Society guidelines for breast screening with MRI as an adjunct to mammography. *CA Cancer J Clin* 57: 75-89, 2007.

26. Gerber DE. Targeted therapies: A new generation of cancer treatments. *Am Fam Physician* 77 (3):311-19, 2008.

27. Offerman M. The era of targeted therapies. *Am Fam Physician* 77 (3):294-5, 2008.

28. Centerwatch. Drugs approved by the FDA, 2007.

29. Ibid #8, p W-45.

30. Abelson R, Pollack A. Medicare widens drugs it accepts for cancer care: More off-label uses. *New York Times*, January 27, 2009: A1.

31. Bennett CL, Silver SM, Djulbegovic B, et al. Venous thromboembolism and mortality associated with recombinant erythropoetin and darbepoetin administration for the treatment of cancer-associated anemia. *JAMA* 299 (8):914-24, 2008.

32. Gryta T. Anemia drugs to carry wider warnings. *Wall Street Journal*, July 31, 2008: B6.

33. Pollack A. Hospitals chase a nuclear tool to fight cancer. *New York Times*, December 26, 2007:A1.

34. Ibid # 33.

35. Pollack A. High-tech cancer fight brings big profit. *New York Times*, December 26, 2007:A22.

36. Ibid #33.

37. Wang X, Yang L, Chen Z, et al. Application of nanotechnology in cancer therapy and imaging. *CA Cancer J Clin* 58: 97-110, 2008.

38. Science & Technology. Treating Tumors: Golden slingshot. *The Economist* 389 (8605), November 8, 2008, pp 97-8.

39. Culliton BJ. Interview. Promoting medical innovation while developing sound social and business policy: A conversation with Thomas G. Roberts. *Health Affairs Web Exclusive* 27 (1): W-34-W35, 2007.

40. Ibid # 39.

41. Pipes SC. *The Top Ten Myths of American Health Care: A Citizens Guide.* San Francisco, CA. PRI. Pacific Research Institute, 2008, p 42.

42. Ibid # 9.

*43.* Butcher L. The high cost of cancer drugs: As treatment bills climb, so does tension between payers and clinicians. *Oncology Times* March 10, 2007: 19

44. Rawlins M. As quoted by Silberman, J., Britain weighs the social cost of high-priced drugs. NPR, July 3, 2008.

45. Ibid # 7.
46. Berenson A. Perverse incentives limit any savings in treating cancer. *New York Times*, July 12, 2007: C1.
47. Chase M. Pricey drugs put squeeze on doctors. *Wall Street Journal,* July 8, 2008: A1.
48. Your health. Prostate cancer. *AARP Bulletin* May, 2008: 16.
49. Evans JP. Health care in the age of genetic medicine. *JAMA* 298 (22): 2670, 2007.
50. Ibid # 8, W-46.

CHAPTER 3

# Cancer Care:
# Priceless, but Can We Afford It?

Assertions that people in the richest country in the world are denied cancer care are often met with disbelief ("We can't be that cruel"); with unrealistic hope ("They'll get care somehow"); with cynicism ("They don't deserve care if they can't pay for it"); or with a plea to a Malthusian view ("It's the same the world over – survival of the fittest"). These beliefs vary in their popularity, but advocates of the current system all proclaim that the marketplace can and will improve access and affordability of cancer care.

Having looked at the size of the cancer problem in Chapter 1, and reviewed in Chapter 2 how our magical bullets of drugs and technology are often backfiring, we now turn to assessing the conditions on the ground. This chapter has two goals: (1) to look at what has been happening to access and affordability of general medical care in the U.S., and (2) to describe and illustrate the special problems facing cancer patients in getting care.

## From Bad to Worse:
## Declining Access and Affordability of Medical Care

Declining access goes hand in hand with surging prices of health care. As is obvious, when prices continue to go up at three or four times the cost of living and median household incomes, access problems grow exponentially worse. All this is happening, with no relief in sight.

Patients and their families are caught in the crosscurrents of three dynamics, the first of which is rising costs. Projected U.S. health expenditures in 2011 totaled $2.7 trillion, $8,649 per capita and 17.7 percent of GDP. By 2020, in spite of the Affordable Care Act, projected health spending is predicted to reach $4.6 trillion, $13,709 per capita and 19.8 percent of GDP.[1]

The second force they confront is a decline in access when they can't afford the care. We will cover the harm resulting from this in depth in a later chapter. In the meantime, here are highlights of what they are facing:

- Despite an increase in government insurance rolls by almost 6 million, the number of uninsured in 2010 surged to 50.7 million.[2]
- According to a 2008 report by the Commonwealth Fund, an additional 25 million are underinsured, up by 60 percent since 2003; 42 percent of adults between 19 and 64 are now uninsured or underinsured.[3]
- Two million cancer patients are foregoing needed care each year due to unaffordable costs.[4]
- A majority of uninsured and underinsured Americans now go without necessary care because of costs (Figure 3.1)[5]
- Lack of access is adversely impacting the health of our population. More than 40 percent of the U.S. population has one or more chronic conditions;[6] those one in six mentioned above who are uninsured are almost four times more likely to go without care than the insured.[7]

The last factor they face is declining ability to pay. The reasons why ability to pay is declining are etched in stark relief by our U.S. economy. Not only are medical costs rising, but:

- 72 million Americans are now having trouble paying their medical bills (41 percent of working-age adults);[8] according to the Center for Studying Health System Change, financial pressures on families from medical bills increase sharply whenever out-of-pocket spending on health care services exceeds 5 percent of family income, or even lower spending levels for low-income families and for people in poor health.[9]
- 64 million Americans under age 65 are in families spending more than 10 percent of their pretax income on health care, according to a recent national study by Families USA; although most have insurance, nearly 19 million spend more than 25 percent of their income on health care.[10]
- One million Americans are bankrupted each year as a result of medical bills. These aren't primarily uninsured or unemployed

FIGURE 3.1

## Underinsured and Uninsured Adults at High Risk of Going Without Needed Care and Financial Stress

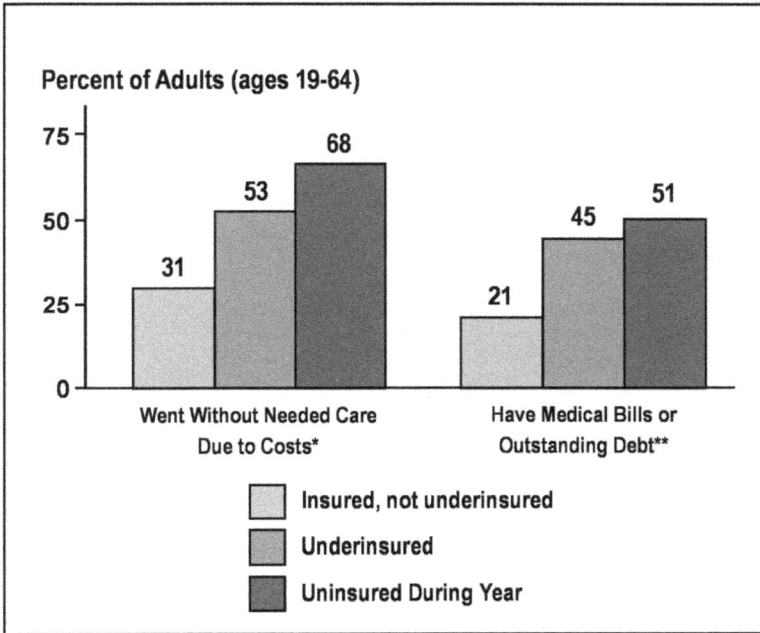

**Percent of Adults (ages 19-64)**

| | Went Without Needed Care Due to Costs* | Have Medical Bills or Outstanding Debt** |
|---|---|---|
| Insured, not underinsured | 31 | 21 |
| Underinsured | 53 | 45 |
| Uninsured During Year | 68 | 51 |

* Did not fill prescription, skipped test, treatment, or follow-up care recommended by a doctor; have a medical problem, but did not visit a doctor; did not get specialist care (at least one of the above)

** Had problem paying medical bills; changed way of life to pay medical bills; contacted by collection agency for bills (any of these)

Source: Reprinted with permission from Schoen C, Collins SR, Krus JL, et al. How many are underinsured? Trends among U.S. adults, 2003 and 2007, *Health Affairs Web Exclusive* June 10, 2008: W298-W309.

people: three out of every four of them were both employed and insured before becoming sick.[11]

• Seniors on fixed incomes are especially hard hit by medical costs; between 1991 and 2007, the bankruptcy filing rate per thousand aged 65 to 74 increased by 125 percent, and for those aged 75 to 84, it skyrocketed by 433 percent.[12]

• Since 1970, the income of the top 0.1 percent of the population has gone up by 385 percent while the income of the bottom 90 percent of us has dropped by 1 percent. [13]

FIGURE 3.2

## The Average Income of the
## Top 5 Percent Has Doubled Since 1980

Household Income in Constant 2005 Dollars

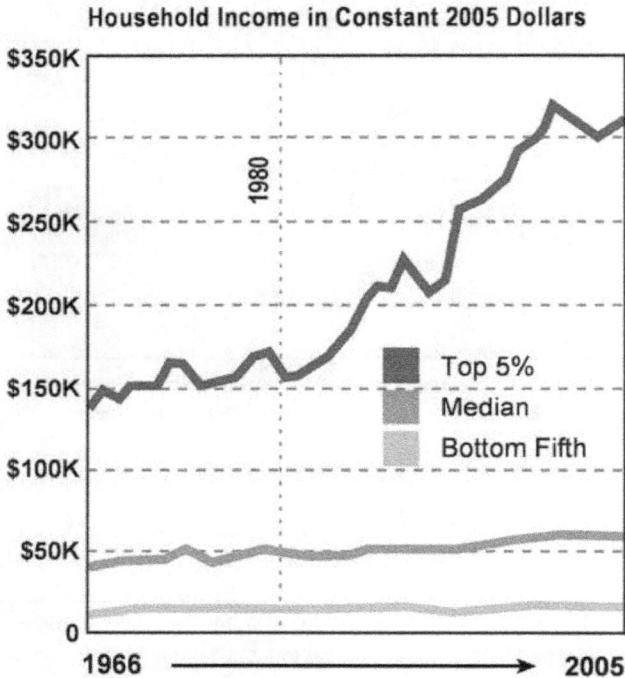

Source: Drucker J. Richest see income share rise. *Wall Street Journal,* July 23, 2008: A3.

- The average income of the top 5 percent of our population has doubled since 1980, while the average income for the other 95 percent has remained stagnant (Figure 3.2).[14]

- Median household debt in 2006 exceeded $100,000, while the median household income was just $41,000 (both as measured in 2000 dollars);[15] the median annual household income today is about $50,000.[16]
- 49 million Americans—16 percent of the population—were living in poverty in 2010. [17]

- The Congressional Budget Office (CBO) reported in late 2008 that workplace retirement plans, including 401(k) plans, have lost $2 trillion in value from mid-2007 to Fall 2008.[18]
- Consumer spending on prescription drugs dropped from 45 percent of dispensed medications in 2003 to 30 percent in 2008, according to IMS Health.[19]
- By the end of 2008, U.S. consumer confidence had fallen to a 40-year low.[20]
- According to a 2008 survey by the *Washington Post*, the Kaiser Family Foundation and Harvard University, of more than 1,300 randomly selected Americans between 18 and 64 years of age who work at least 30 hours a week and earn less than $27,000 a year, 8 of 10 found it difficult to pay for gasoline and other transportation costs or save money for retirement, while 7 out of 10 found it difficult to afford health insurance.[21]

These realities reveal not the market-based cornucopia constantly promised by advocates of the current system, but an increasingly barren wilderness where families are left to fend for themselves with fewer and fewer resources with which to cope.

These three interrelated forces of skyrocketing costs, decreasing access, and a decline in the ability to pay for health care might once have been blunted by unemployment benefits. But as unemployment rates rise, a majority of people losing their jobs no longer qualify for unemployment benefits, which are being further threatened by Republicans' austerity efforts. More than one in four people applying for unemployment compensation now have their benefit claims disputed by employers and state agencies.[22] The national average of those receiving these benefits fell from 55 percent in 1958 to 44 percent in 2001 and only 37 percent in 2008, according to the Labor Department.[23] Women are especially hard hit by our economic downturn as a result of outsourcing, layoffs and stagnant wages.[24] These forces make a mockery of those who allege that people do without insurance as a matter of choice.

Life choices are also being impacted at both ends of working careers for men and women. Many couples are moving wedding dates up to enroll both husband and wife on a company's health insurance plan. Or couples may delay a divorce in order to retain their insurance coverage.[25] Many families have refinanced their homes in order to pay for high medical care costs, such as surgery and other cancer treatments. But falling housing prices have now blocked refinancing as a method of paying medical bills for huge sectors of the population.[26] Meanwhile, one in four people between 45 and 54 years of age plan to delay retirement because of the economy. And a late 2008 projection by the Bureau of Labor estimates that the number of people over 65 in the labor pool will grow by 74 percent by 2014.[27] Though they will then have Medicare, many will still struggle to pay the costs of care that Medicare does not cover, which amount to about one-half of their total costs.[28]

## Cancer Care: Even Greater Financial Worries

Difficult as it is for much of our population to gain access to affordable health care today, access is much more difficult for patients with cancer, even as they deal with a life-threatening disease. The costs of cancer care, as we have already seen glimpses of, are going through the roof at rates much above those for general medical care. According to a recent study by researchers at the University of Minnesota, Ovation Pharmaceuticals raised prices on four of its drugs by up to 3,436 percent (not a typo!) in 2006. The ethics of the market were laid bare when one of these drugs targeted for that maximal price increase was Cosmegen, a drug used for Wilms' tumor, a cancer of the kidney in children. Note the dynamic: Markets promise plummeting prices in theory. Yet here, because of patents and high development costs that minimize competition, combined with little or no regulation of pricing, "market-based medicine" means the sky is the limit.[29]

Three approved targeted drugs for cancer now cost about $100,000 a year.[30] Other cancer care services are not far behind in their costs. A course of proton beam therapy for cancer of the prostate, discussed in Chapter Two, costs $50,000,[31] each robotic surgery procedure for that cancer consumes $1,500 to $2,000 in disposable instruments and accessories,[32] and each PET imaging procedure costs about $2,000.

In many instances, manufacturers and suppliers are free to set their own prices. Unlike commodities priced at whatever the market will bear, cancer treatments have a different spin on the price: your money or your life is often the only choice patients and their families face. Hospitals typically pass these costs along to insurers, who in turn pass them back to patients in higher premiums. Patients and their families usually see little recourse but to try to cope with these prices in hopes of therapeutic benefits.

Here are various ways by which cancer patients have special problems in gaining access to essential cancer care today.

## No Insurance

This is unfortunately a big and widespread problem. As already noted, one-sixth of our population is uninsured. One-third of people under 65 who are diagnosed with cancer are uninsured during or after diagnosis, with three of four reporting their lack of coverage due to unaffordable premium costs or a pre-existing condition exclusion.[33] The Institute of Medicine has found that 11 percent of cancer survivors between 25 and 64 years of age are uninsured. Younger cancer survivors (25 to 44) are more often uninsured (19 percent) than their counterparts who have never had cancer, as are Hispanic/Latino cancer survivors (26 percent). Thus we have a system in which those who need insurance the most – survivors of cancer who face higher instances of recurrence than the general population – are less likely to have insurance than are people who haven't had cancer.[34]

Even if insured, cancer patients are vulnerable to losing their jobs and their insurance, as this patient's experience illustrates:

> *Lori, 51, is a survivor from breast cancer. After a nine-month period of treatment during which she was unable to work, she is now strapped for money and needs to go back to work. But she is afraid to admit to potential employers the reason for her nine-month gap in her work record, fearing that her history of cancer will work against her. As she says, "It's like I'm hiding something awful because I got sick."*[35]

Lori's problem is common. A 2009 study of more than 20,000 cancer survivors in the U.S. and Europe found that they are 37 percent more likely to be unemployed than their healthier peers.[36]

Cancer survivors younger than 65 without Medicare report not getting needed care (44 percent) or filling needed prescriptions (31 percent).[37] A 2007 study by the Kaiser Family Foundation and the Harvard School of Public Health found that almost one-half of cancer patients without consistent health insurance during their course of treatment used up all or most of their savings and had no money for basic necessities.[38]

This patient's experience illustrates the difficult circumstances that uninsured people with cancer face.

> *Susan, 46, of Asheville, North Carolina was self-employed without insurance when she was found to have liposarcoma in 2003. She cashed out her 401(k) plan and turned that money over to a hospital in order to qualify for Medicaid by spending down her assets. Although she did gain Medicaid coverage, she still had $20,000 in hospital bills not covered by Medicaid, and her debts kept increasing because of out-of-pocket expenses. In 2007 she refinanced her home to cut her debts down to $28,000, but in 2008 she had surgery to remove cancer from her lung. As she grimly acknowledges, "I will once again be cancer free, but over my head in debt. There's no more money (equity) in my house to mortgage it again."*[39]

## Can't Get Insurance

As a 2006 report of the Institute of Medicine pointed out, people with any history of cancer are usually denied insurance coverage. Cancer survivors attempting to buy insurance face three kinds of barriers – availability, affordability, and adequacy.[40] Even when insurance can be found, it comes at high cost for very limited coverage. Figure 3.3 compares the cumulative change in health insurance premiums with federal poverty levels from 1996 to 2004.[41] The average premium for employer-sponsored insurance for a family of four hit $15,073 in 2011, with employees paying $4,129 of that, and average annual employee premium costs are expected to go up by another 10.6 percent in 2012.[42,43]

Cancer patients are especially vulnerable to increases. For them, such increases in the costs of health insurance come at a time of huge financial drain: large co-pays, often unpaid leave from work due to illness, diminished income for caregivers who may also be taking time off work. In short, increased premiums that would be a hardship for many healthy families become devastating for cancer patients.

## Have Insurance, But Coverage Denied

Even with insurance, insurers can go to great lengths to deny payment for cancer care, as illustrated by this patient's experience.

*Adrian, 19, was a college student with insurance through General Motors with BlueCross BlueShield of Michigan. Her physician found pre-cancerous cells on her Pap smear and advised her to have three shots of Guardasil, the HPV vaccine. The insurer refused payment for the vaccine on the grounds that it was still experimental, not yet approved by the FDA. Four years later, at 23, she was found to have cervical cancer requiring surgery. Again, BCBS denied coverage (about $6,000), this time on the basis of a Michigan law forbidding operations on a woman's reproductive system under the age of 26. As shown*

FIGURE 3.3

## Cumulative Changes in Health Insurance Premiums, Overall Inflation, and Workers' Earnings, 2000-2007

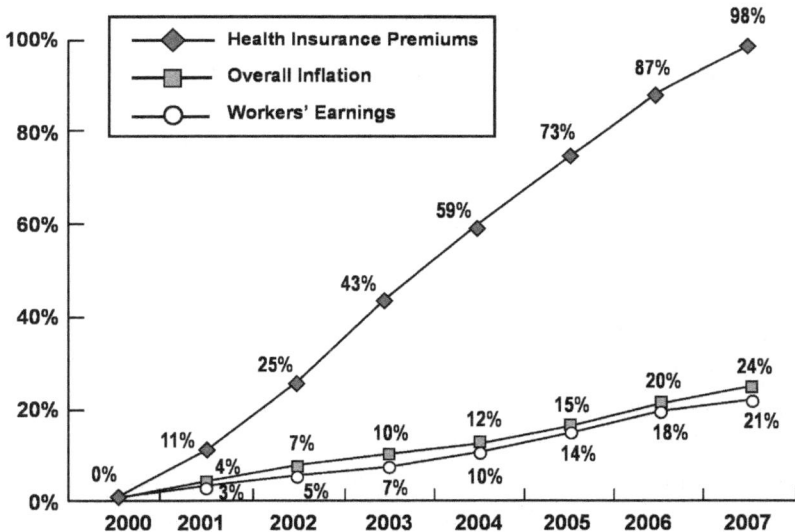

*Source: Kaiser Family Foundation. Snapshots: Health Care Costs. Effect of tying eligibility for health insurance subsidies to the federal poverty level. February 2007.*

*\* Reprinted with permission from the Henry J. Kaiser Family Foundation. The Kaiser Family Foundation is a non-profit private operating foundation, based in Menlo Park, California, dedicated to producing and communicating the best possible information, research and analysis on health issues.*

*in Michael Moore's film SICKO, Adrian traveled to Canada, where she had surgery a few days after the diagnosis.*[44]

## Insurance Cancelled

*Patsy, 52, was in the midst of chemotherapy for breast cancer when her coverage by Health Net was cancelled. The company claimed that she had not disclosed a heart condition and had incorrectly listed her weight on her initial application for insurance. A Health Net broker had completed the application for Patsy, and had later changed her reported weight from 185 to 165 pounds. In January 2004, the company cancelled her policy, stating that she would have been denied coverage initially based on her actual weight. Patsy was left with $129,000 in medical bills and had to stop chemotherapy for several months until she found a charity to pay for it. Four years later, a private arbitration judge found Health Net's conduct and cancellation policies "reprehensible", and ordered Health Net to pay more than $9 million in compensation to Patsy.*[45-47]

Patsy was the victim of a common tactic used by private insurers to avoid paying expensive claims and pad their financial bottom line. They typically defend these cancellations on the alleged failure of enrollees to fully disclose their history on their initial application for insurance or how applicants had answered questions that are often vague or confusing.

This conflict is not merely the difference of opinion between the insurance company and the insured. Something far more systematic is taking place. Blue Cross of California, now owned by Wellpoint, the nation's largest private health insurer, was fined $1 million by a state regulator in 2006 for cancelling policies.[48] Health Net Inc., another large for-profit insurer in California, had a policy setting monthly targets for cancellations. They tied this target to staff bonuses. One senior analyst cancelled 1,600 policies between 2000 and 2006, receiving $20,000 in bonuses. The California Department of Managed Health Care also fined Health Net $1 million for this practice.[49]

## Increasing Co-Payments

*Julie, 52, has metastatic breast cancer. She lives on Social Security disability payments. Because of her disability status,*

*she has coverage through a Medicare HMO. As her disease ad-
vances, her physician prescribes Tykerb, a Tier 4 drug, which
she can't afford. As she says, "For everybody in my position
with metastatic breast cancer, there are times when you are stable and can go off treatment... But if you are progressing, we
have to be on treatment, or we will die... People's eyes need to
be opened. They need to understand that these drugs are very
costly, and that there are a lot of people out there who are struggling with these costs."*[50]

Insurers in the past have charged small co-payments, such as $20
to $30 for each prescription drug, That time has long since passed for
many drugs, especially chemotherapy and anti-anemia drugs commonly
used in cancer treatment. As the costs of these drugs soar out of sight,
insurers try to keep premiums down for employers by charging patients
much higher co-payments – now often 20 to 33 percent of the drug
costs. Insurers have adopted systems to "tier" drugs by class and cost
of drugs. Tier 4 drugs are the most expensive, including such drugs
as Procrit for anemia and Neupogen for immuno-suppressed patients.
The resulting co-payments can be devastating for patients. Examples
include: $13,500 for a 90-day supply of a drug for chronic myelogenous
leukemia, $3,480 for a 21-day supply of Tykerb for metastatic breast
cancer.[51]

Both health economists and patients are alarmed by these costs.
James Robinson, Ph.D., well-known health economist at the University
of California Berkeley, calls this financing mechanism "very poor
social policy... This new system sticks seriously ill people with huge
bills... This is an erosion of the traditional concept of insurance."[52]

**Cash and Carry**

As they confront burgeoning bad-debt and charity-care costs, many
U.S. hospitals are requiring patients to pay large cash payments up front
before they are admitted to the hospital. According to the American
Hospital Association, uncompensated care cost the hospital industry
over $32 billion in 2006. This is up 44 percent from 2000. These
levels of bad debt, of course, are driven by high prices of hospital care,
growing numbers of uninsured and underinsured patients, and higher
deductibles and co-payments making it more difficult for patients to
pay hospitals.

That large investor-owned hospital chains, such as HCA and Tenet, impose rigorous requirements for cash up front comes as no surprise. But a growing number of "not-for-profit" hospitals have also taken up this policy and have themselves become big businesses. The well-known M .D. Anderson Cancer Center in Houston is one such example. It operates as a tax-exempt facility under the state university system in Texas, with only 6 percent of its budget coming from the state. As a leading cancer center, it generates large profits and attracts sizable philanthropic donations. In 2007, it had a net income of $310 million; its cash, investments, and endowments now total almost $1.9 billion. Yet despite these prodigious resources, its free care has been falling off. This is one patient's harrowing experience in gaining admission to the hospital.

> *Lisa, 52, was diagnosed with acute leukemia in late 2006, and her physician referred her to M. D. Anderson for urgent care. On arrival at the hospital, she was told that she would need to pay $105,000 before she could be admitted. Lisa had a limited benefit policy through UnitedHealth, but the hospital would not accept her insurance and viewed her as uninsured. She was next told that she could get an appointment if she brought in a certified check for $45,000. Although Lisa and her husband lived comfortably and owned an apartment building and a rental house, they didn't have that amount of cash on hand. Her husband borrowed the money from his father's trust, and she returned to the hospital, where she had blood drawn and a bone marrow biopsy performed. Her oncologist wanted to admit her right away, but the hospital then demanded an additional $60,000 as a down payment for her treatment, saying that the $45,000 was just for the laboratory tests. The hospital later reduced that requirement to $30,000 and Lisa was admitted, after some hours, as an "override" admission.*
>
> *After 8 days in the hospital, Lisa was discharged with a plan for chemotherapy for more than a year. The hospital still expected up front payments for her appointments, which were sometimes "blocked" – until she made payments at the Business Office. On one day, the nurses wouldn't change her chemotherapy bag, which beeped for an hour until her husband returned from the Business Office with proof of payment. Despite these*

*obstacles, Lisa was still in chemotherapy at M.D. Anderson in May of 2008. UnitedHealth had paid $38,478 toward her medical bills. She changed over to a BlueCross BlueShield policy, which covers more of her bills, but still had more than $145,000 in outstanding bills, which she is paying down by $2,000 a month. Having been in remission for more than a year, her leukemia has returned, and her saga continues. The hospital is giving her a 10 percent discount on her balance, but only if she pays $130,640 within a few days.*[53]

## Increasing Credit Card Debt

Credit card debt for medical bills is growing at a rapid rate. CMS projects that patients' out-of-pocket (OOP) spending for medical care to rise from $269 billion in 2007 to $464 billion by 2017. Extending credit for this purpose has recently become big business. GE Money Care Credit and ChaseHealthAdvance are two such examples of these new credit plans. Lenders' cuts of physicians' fees can be as high as 13.5 percent, and interest rates for patients can reach 27.99 percent. These plans serve the interests of hospitals and other providers, whether or not they are in their patients' advantage, and 31 state medical and veterinarian associations and 11 other national groups have endorsed the concept. Some $45 billion of medical expenses are charged now on credit cards, and that amount is expected to more than triple by 2015. Claudia Lennhoff, executive director of Champaign County Health Care Consumers, a nonprofit consumer health advocacy organization in Champaign, Illinois, has this to say about this new trend:

> "The consumers who come to us for help when they are struggling with CareCredit debt are desperate people who were required to provide payment for an appendectomy or cancer treatment at the time of service. Health care providers steered them into these finance plans with rates that they didn't understand. This is really the medical equivalent of sub-prime mortgages."[54]

## Exclusions of Out-of-Pocket (OOP) Limits

Out-of-pocket costs are typically very high, much higher than anticipated, for almost all patients with cancer. A 2008 survey by the National Medical Expenditure Panel found that more than 13 percent of non-elderly patients with cancer spent at least 20 percent of their income on health care and insurance. More than four in ten patients with individual health insurance spent over 20 percent of their incomes on medical expenses. [55]

Many insurers offer the financial protections to enrollees of OOP limits to their spending over a year, especially for such services as physician visits and hospital stays. But the high costs of chemotherapy drugs are often excluded (in fine print) from OOP limits. The General Accounting Office has found that about one-third of Medicare Advantage plans, if they offer any OOP limits as all, exclude spending on Part B drugs – chemotherapy and others such as anti-anemia drugs. Patients are often unaware of these exclusions until they need them. Florida-based WellCare, for example, advertises an annual OOP limit of $3,750 in its "Concert" Medicare Advantage plan. However, the Medicare Rights Center learned that chemotherapy drugs are specifically excluded from the OOP limit on page 155 of the WellCare Evidence of Coverage document.[56]

**Breaking Through Lifetime Coverage Limits**

As has been mentioned in an earlier chapter, many private insurers impose lifetime caps on coverage for enrollees, typically at about $2 million. While that might first appear to give a patient protection against future health expenses, such caps are increasingly becoming a serious threat to a growing number of patients with chronic illnesses as costs of care continue skyward. The Kaiser Family Foundation has found that 55 percent of workers with employer-sponsored insurance had lifetime limits in 2007, including 23 percent with caps less than $2 million.[57] As public awareness of this new problem grows, legislation to raise these lifetime caps becomes a policy option, which is of course opposed by the insurance industry. These two patients' experiences show how precarious even a $2 million lifetime cap can be, and how quickly it can be reached.

> • *Karlin, 43, fully employed and insured as assistant manager of Sam Goody at the Deptford Mall in Philadelphia, was diagnosed with acute myeloid leukemia in 2007. Over the next 16 months, her insurance covered chemotherapy, a bone marrow transplant, and five months in hospitals. But then her insurer notified her that she had reached her lifetime cap of $2 million, and she became uninsured. UnitedHealthcare, as the*

*parent company for her insurer, defended this action in this way: "The primary reason – for caps is to lower the cost of insurance so employers can cover as many people as possible." But Gary Claxton, health policy expert at the Kaiser Family Foundation, counters that: "What insurance is supposed to do best is handle the extraordinary thing that is rare. So to some extent, these policies are not protecting the people who most need insurance. These people did everything they were supposed to do. They were paying their premiums, insurance companies are finding ways to limit exposure of these policies to really sick people."*[58]

*...*

• *Deb, 41, was diagnosed with acute lymphoblastic leuke-mia (ALL) in 2005. Over the first year and a half of care, her costs exceeded $1 million, including a month in the hospital for a stem cell transplant, five five-day hospital stays for inpatient chemotherapy (each costing $137,000), a four-day stay for total body radiation, a three-week hospitalization for encephalitis, another week for bronchitis, and a week for neurological test-ing.*

*Deb was fortunate to have employer-sponsored insurance. She was no longer able to work, received COBRA, became eli-gible for disability through Social Security, together with long-term disability at $100 per month through her former employer. Deb and her daughter moved home with her parents to save money, but her financial challenges remained. Her insurance premium went up by 150 percent in January 2008, she owes money to six hospitals, and her co-payments for medications for graft-vs.-host disease can come to $900 a month. She often tries to save money by skipping some of her medication doses, and fears breaking through the $2 million lifetime cap someday. As she says: "I pray every day that I never relapse, not because of the death thing, but because I know I can't afford it."*[59]

## A Fragile Safety Net

One might assume that there will be a safety net when the costs of care become overwhelming. But that assumption is unrealistic. Whatever safety net we once had is rapidly falling apart.

As is now common knowledge, 2.6 million jobs were lost during

2008 in this country, including 524,000 lost in December alone. The unemployment rate is at a 16-year high.60 You may expect that COBRA will help. This is the government program established by the Consolidated Omnibus Budget Reconciliation Act of 1985, under which a newly unemployed person may continue group health insurance, if previously insured through the employer, for a period up to 18 months. But many unemployed, even if having had employer-sponsored insurance, find the costs of COBRA coverage (100 percent of the costs of premiums plus a 2 percent administrative charge), prohibitively expensive. A January 2009 report by the Bureau of Labor Statistics and the Agency for Healthcare Research and Quality found that average COBRA premiums come to $1,069 a month and swallow up 83.6 percent of their entire unemployment income.61 A 2009 report by the Commonwealth Fund found that only 9 percent of jobless workers actually continue coverage under COBRA.62 Given the costs, this finding is no surprise.

Medicaid is also a tenuous part of the safety net as it continues to unravel under the pressure of federal and state deficits. You have to prove that you are destitute before you can become eligible for Medicaid. A 2007 study by Public Citizen's Health Research Group found that 60 percent of poor Americans are not covered by Medicaid.63 Eligibility and coverage policies vary widely from state to state; in Missouri, a family of three with an annual income of $3,504 a year (less than one-quarter of the federal poverty level) exceeds the eligibility threshold. If one transfers assets in an attempt to qualify for Medicaid, eligibility will be delayed for a period of time (e.g. if Medicaid pays $150 a day for nursing home care, you'll be ineligible for 666 days if you give away $100,000 in assets (the math arriving at 666 days being $100,000 divided by $150).64 By 2011, many states were making draconian cuts in Medicaid coverage; as examples, California has eliminated adult day care coverage and limits patients to seven physician visits a year, while Hawaii plans to limit Medicaid hospital coverage to just 10 days a year starting in 2012. 65

## So Where Does This Leave Us?

What do all these costs and various situations tell us about whether we will be able to afford cancer care? Throughout this chapter we have focused on the predicaments patients face, from inadequate insurance to demands for upfront payments that they can't afford. While harrowing in the details, it is worth remembering our focus: Are we deploying our resources to most effectively deal with cancer, a very large problem for the country? Looked at from that perspective, the tragedies described in this chapter, while exacting their individual toll, also reveal a massive diversion of resources – taking away from patients and placing them into the hands of insurers, providers and lenders.

It may be tempting to think that the dynamic of rising costs and lowered care will continue indefinitely, and that somehow patients, insurers or the government will just keep paying for it. After all, medical care, regardless of cost, is a necessity. But just as it was once popular to believe equity in homes would rise forever and people would pay any price to own a home, only to see that bubble burst, so we may see a bubble collapse in medical costs. As with housing, the fallout will be ugly, with widespread and unexpected casualties.

Wall Street analysts are already seeing evidence that the bubble is contracting. As an example, Johnson & Johnson, the world's largest health care products maker, is warned investors to expect that 2009 would bring its first revenue decline in 76 years; its pharmaceuticals unit had an 11 percent drop in revenue in the fourth quarter of 2008, as a result of our recession with layoffs, loss of drug coverage, and higher copayments.66 Moreover, the annual number of patient visits to physicians dropped by more than 12 percent between 2008 and 2010. 67

Later chapters will focus on what we can do about our growing problem in affording cancer care. We will also ask whether we should abandon the private health insurance industry altogether and replace it with a single-payer financing system, Medicare for All, coupled with a private delivery system. But for now we need to move to the next chapter to ask: what are the prerequisites for availability of effective cancer care for all?

# References

1.  Office of the Actuary, CMS, National Health Spending Projections Through 2020, Health Affairs, July 28, 2011.
2.  Abrons, H. What if everyone had Medicare? San Francisco Chronicle, September 24, 2010.

3.  Schoen C, Collins SR, Krus JL, et al. How many are underinsured? Trends among U.S. adults, 2003 and 2007, Health Affairs Web Exclusive June 10, 2008: W298-W309.

4.  Weaver, KE, Roland, JH, Bellizzi, KM, Ariz, NM. Foregoing medical care because of cost: Assessing disparities in healthcare access among cancer survivors living in the United States. Cancer online, June 14, 2010.

5.  Ibid # 3.

6.  Hoffman C, Schwartz K. Eroding access among nonelderly U.S. adults with chronic conditions: Ten years of change. Health Affairs Web Exclusive, July 22, 2008.

7.  Wilber AP, Woolhandler S, Lasser KE, et al. A national study of chronic disease prevalence and access to care in uninsured U.S. adults. Ann Intern Med 149: 170-6, 2008.

8.  Collins SR, Kriss JL, Doty MM et al. Losing ground: How the loss of adequate health insurance is burdening working families. Commonwealth Fund, Volume 99, August 20, 2008.

9.  Cunningham PJ, Miller C, Cassil A. Living on the edge: Health care expenses strain family budgets. Center for Studying Health System Change. Washington, D.C., December, 2008.

10. Lazar K., High healthcare costs taking toll on insured. The Boston Globe, May 2, 2009.

11. Himmelstein DU, Warren E, Thorne D, et al. Illness and injury as contributors to bankruptcy. Health Affairs Web Exclusive W5-63, 2005.

12. Associated Press. Bankruptcies rise for older set. Wall Street Journal, August 28, 2008: D6.

13. Rothschild, M. Enlist for class warfare. The Progressive, September 20, 2011.

14. Spriggs WE. The economic crisis in black and white. American Prospect 19 (10): A3, October, 2008.

15. Henderson N. Greenspan's mixed legacy: America prospered during the Fed chief's tenure, but built up massive debt. Washington Post National Weekly Edition, January 30-February 5, 2006, p 6.

16. U.S. Census Bureau. Census Bureau releases 2009 American Community Survey data. September 28, 2010.

17. Fletcher, MA. Census Bureau measures more Americans living in poverty. The Washington Post, November 7, 2011.

18. Levitz J. Workplace retirement plans suffer $2 trillion in losses. Wall Street Journal, October 8, 2008: D2.

19. Wang SS, Johnson A. Patients curb prescription spending. Wall Street Journal, July 16, 2008: B1.

20. Grynbaum MM. Consumer confidence, battered by market setbacks, sags to a 40-year low. New York Times October 29, 2008: B7.

21. Fletcher MA, Cohen J. Barely making it. Low-wage workers hover just above poverty, yet keep grasping for the American dream. Washington Post National Weekly Edition, August 11-17, 2008: 22-4.

22. Whoriskey P. Out of work and challenged on benefits: Employers are moving

in record numbers to block unemployment benefits. Washington Post National Weekly Edition, February 16-22, 2009: 24.

23. Troianovski A. Majority of jobless in U.S. don't get benefits. Wall Street Journal, July 28, 2008: A4.
24. Uchitelle L. Women are now equal as victims of poor economy. New York Times, July 22, 2008: A1.
25. Knight VE. Anxiety over health insurance shapes life choices. Wall Street Journal, June 10, 2008: D2.
26. Rubenstein S. Facing a choice between home and health care. Wall Street Journal, November 25, 2008: D1.
27. Fleck C. Retirement on hold. AARP Bulletin 49(6): 10, 2008.
28. Moon M. Will the care be there? Vulnerable beneficiaries and Medicare reform. Health Affairs (Millwood) 18: 107-17, 1999.
29. Appleby J. Drug prices up 100% -- or higher. USA Today, August 8-10, 2008: 1A.
30. McKoy JM, Fitzner KA, Edwards BJ, et al. Cost considerations in the management of cancer in the older patient. Oncology 21 (7): 852, 2007.
31. Pollack A. Hospitals chase a nuclear tool to fight cancer. New York Times, December 26, 2007: A1.
32. Alpert B. Robot dreams. Barrons July 28, 2008, accessed on line at http://online.barrons.com/article_print/SB121702598388786149.html?mod=b_hps_9_0001... 7/28/2008.
33. American Cancer Society. A national poll: Facing cancer in the health care system, 2010.
34. Hewitt M, Greenfield S, Stovall E, eds. From Cancer Patient to Survivor: Lost in Transition. Washington, DC. The National Academies Press, 2006: p 11.
35. Rabin RC. Joblessness risk found high among cancer survivors. New York Times, February 18, 2009: A15.
36. deBoer AGEM, Taskila T, Ojajarvi A, et al. Cancer survivors and unemployment. JAMA 301 (7): 753-62, 2009.
37. Ibid # 34.
38. Eastman P. New survey confirms high cost of cancer in U.S. families. Oncology Today January 10: 4.
39. Ibid # 26.
40. Ibid # 32.
41. Kaiser Family Foundation. Snapshots: Health Care Costs. Effect of tying eligibility for health insurance subsidies to the federal poverty level. February, 2007.
42. Appleby, J. Costs of employer insurance plans surge in 2011. Kaiser Health News, September 27, 2011.
43. Japsen, B. Companies pass on more of health costs to workers. New York Times, October 3, 2011.
44. Burns M. Bad faith by insurers is bad health care. The Progressive Populist 14 (1): 11, 2008.
45. Girion L. Health Net ordered to pay $9 million after cancelling cancer patient's policy. Los Angeles Times, February 23, 2008.

46. AARP. In the News. Cancer patient awarded millions. AARP Bulletin 49 (3): 4, 2008.

47. Case No.: BC321432. Interim Arbitration Award (Binding). Patsy Bates vs. Health Net Inc. et al. By Sam Cianchetti, Judge, (retired).

48. Girion L. The nation. Blue Cross settling patients' lawsuits. The big insurer, accused of illegally canceling some policies, agrees to pay its ex-customers. Los Angeles Times, October 18, 2006:A1.

49. Medicare Rights Center. California-based insurance plan fined $1million. New York: Medicare Watch 10 (24): November 27, 2007.

50. Kolata G. Co-payments go way up for drugs with high costs. Insurers shift burden. New York Times, April 14, 2008: A1.

51. Ibid # 50.

52. Ibid # 50

53. Martinez B. Cash before chemo: Hospitals get tough. Wall Street Journal, April 28, 2008: A1.

54. Consumer Reports. CR Investigates. Overdose of debt: Lenders push risky credit for everything from cancer care to Botox. Consumer Reports July, 2009, pp 14-18.

55. Bernard, DSM, Farr, SL, Fang, Z. National estimates of out-of-pocket health care expenditure burdens among non-elderly adults with cancer: 2001 to 2008. Journal of Clinical Oncology, June 2011.

56. Medicare Rights Center. Sticking it to patients. Asclepios, August 7, 2008.

57. Lee C. More hitting cost limits on health benefits. Washington Post, January, 27, 2008: A.

58. Vitez M. Fairness of insurance caps is questioned. The Philadelphia Inquirer, December 15, 2008.

59. Personal communication, January 6, 2008.

60. Freking K. Health coverage goes with jobs. Associated Press. January 10, 2009.

61. Graham J. COBRA unaffordable for most families. Triage. Chicago Tribune, January 9, 2009.

62. McQueen MP. Jobless can't afford to extend health coverage. Wall Street Journal, January 24, 2009: B2.

63. Public Citizen. Unsettling scores: A ranking of State Medicaid programs. Health Letter 23 (4): April, 2007.

64. Solomon D. Wrestling with Medicaid cuts. Wall Street Journal, February 16, 2006: A4.

65. Galewitz, P. States are limiting Medicaid hospital coverage in search of savings. Kaiser Health News, October 24, 2011.

66. Loftus, P, Wang, SS. J & J sales show health care feels the pinch. Wall Street Journal, February 16, 2006: A4.

67. Johnson, A, Rockoff, JD, Mathews, AW. Americans cut back on visits to doctor. Wall Street Journal, July 29, 2010:A1.

CHAPTER 4

# Prerequisites for Availability of Effective Cancer Care But Can We Afford It?

"We are now at a point where the money spent worldwide for a single drug will exceed the entire budget of the National Cancer Institute. We could not have dreamed of this a few years ago. This is not tenable, even for the wealthiest country in the world, let alone for other countries."[1]

—Kevin J. Cullen, M.D.
Director, University of Maryland Greenebaum Cancer Center

"Society will need to decide what it is willing to pay for quality-adjusted years of life. That decision can be driven by a logical approach or set of standards similar to what has been done in assessing the 'value' of screening tests for cancers, or it can be done by default by insurance denials and the continued evolution toward a two-tiered standard for medical care."[2]

—Frank L. Meyskens, Jr., M.D.
Director, Chao Family Comprehensive Cancer Center
University of California Irvine Medical Center[2]

The above observations by leading oncologists call attention to the increasing stakes and unsustainability of cost trends in cancer care. As we saw in the last chapter, the biggest challenge is to make cancer care affordable to all of those unfortunate enough to get cancer. Standing in the way are market forces that continue unchecked as they drive costs upward well beyond the costs of living and people's ability to afford care. These costs pose an enormous challenge to the cancer community's ability to provide care.

But there are other serious problems that also need to be addressed if we are to keep up with our population's need for essential care.

Resolution of these problems is critical to enabling our delivery system to meet the nation's expanding needs for cancer care. This chapter briefly describes six of these problems.

## 1. We have a declining capacity to meet a growing need for cancer care.

As we have already seen in Chapter 1, older people are at higher risk for cancer, and our aging population carries with it a big increase in the prevalence of cancer. Figure 1.2 reminds us of the extent of this increase. One in five Americans will be 65 or older by 2036. By 2050, the number of Americans 65 and older with cancer will double, while that number will quadruple for those over 85.[3] Four out of ten Americans can expect to be diagnosed with cancer at some point in their lives.[4] Within the next 10 years, cancer will replace heart disease as the number one cause of death in the U.S.[5]

Beyond these numbers, however, care for older cancer patients is much more complex and challenging than is care for younger patients with cancer. Older patients are likely, almost certain, to have multiple co-morbidities, especially heart disease, diabetes, arthritis, dementia, or other functional impairments of one kind or another. From screening to treatment and follow-up, their care needs to be carefully individualized and take into account co-morbidities, health status, quality of life, psychosocial issues, and life expectancy.

In his 1988 Presidential address to the American Society of Clinical Oncology (ASCO), Dr. B. J. Kennedy laid out the future challenge for cancer care in these terms:

> "...our society need not ration how we will treat our disadvantaged members, but should continue to seek those preventive and positive measures that can shorten our later period of morbidity (being sick). A very major cancer load will persist well into the 21st century, even if the attempts at prevention are eventually a total success. There is a developing knowledge on aging. Care of the older person needs to be part of medical education and oncology education. Research will help attain a desirable quality of life with aging and a reduced morbidity."[6]

More than twenty years have elapsed since that warning, yet we are still way behind the curve in meeting these new demands. Oncologists recognize that, more than ever, a team approach to prevention, diagnosis and management of cancer is required. But our primary care infrastructure, upon which continuity of comprehensive care depends, is deteriorating rapidly. As a result of a large gap between procedure-based reimbursement of physician services and the more time-intensive services of physicians in family medicine, general internal medicine, and geriatrics, young physicians are flocking to higher-reimbursed specialties with more attractive life styles. This results in an increasing mal-distribution of physicians by specialty. No more than 8 percent of U.S. medical graduates select family medicine today, with just two percent of those entering internal medicine wanting to be general internists. [7,8] These specialties from which graduates are fleeing are the very foundation of prevention and early diagnosis, as well as coordinated and comprehensive medical care. Specialists in non-primary care fields, including oncology, are ill prepared by training, practice style, or motivation to provide primary care.[9]

In short, we should be gearing up to meet an increasing need, yet instead are running in the opposite direction.

**2. Access is declining while disparities are increasing.**

That the continuing escalation of health care costs makes care less affordable and lowers access is obvious. But even if costs could be contained, as appears impossible in the current marketplace, there are still many barriers to care in this country that lead to marked health disparities within our population. These include insurance status, socioeconomic factors, racial and ethnic differences, cultural and language barriers, risk factors and co-morbidities.

These health disparities are striking and shameful for a wealthy country with such advanced resources for cancer care. The highlights of this hall of shame include:

- Cancer mortality rates are 35 percent higher for African-Americans than whites.[10]
- African American men have a 25 percent higher cancer incidence and 43 percent higher mortality rate from all cancers combined than Caucasian men.[11]
- Although African American women have lower incidence rates than do Caucasian women for all cancers combined, they have a 20 percent higher mortality rate.[12]

- Caucasian women are up to 29 percent more likely than black women to have breast cancer, but African American women are 28 percent more likely to die of their disease.[13]
- American Indians and Alaska Natives have the worst survival from all cancers combined for all racial and ethnic groups.[14]
- In an era that has seen the election of our first African-American president, it would be easy to believe that these disparities are on the decline. But a 2008 study by the American Cancer Society found that black-white disparities from cancers potentially affected by screening and treatment have increased over most time periods since 1975.[15]
- How big a problem are these disparities? According to a 2008 report from the World Health Organization, 886,202 deaths could have been prevented between 1991 and 2000 if access to medical care for African-Americans was equal to that of Caucasians.[16]

All this has led Dr. Antonia Novello, former U.S. Surgeon General, to this conclusion:

"People of color have experienced inequality in health status and health care in the United States for over 200 years. In the 21st century, despite tremendous advances in medicine, the health of minority people has not edged significantly closer to that of the majority... such disparities and catastrophes in the lives of minorities are tolerated because they are overwhelmingly disparities of poor people. The aura of inevitability or even failure that has surrounded disparities for so many decades is perpetuated today by indifference on the part of the majority and loss of hope on the part of the minority."[17]

Insurance status is clearly a major determinant of access to care. The uninsured, of course, have great difficulty affording cancer care. The Institute of Medicine has found that 11 percent of cancer survivors between 25 and 64 years of age are uninsured; within this group 51 percent delay getting medical care, 44 percent don't get needed care, and 31 percent report not filling prescriptions.[18] If one expects that Medicaid will serve as a safety net for these patients, that is unlikely. Eligibility and coverage requirements vary widely from state to state;

virtually all states are facing deficits and many are cutting back on eligibility and Medicaid benefits. In Nevada, for example, state cutbacks have recently forced the only public hospital in Las Vegas to shut down its outpatient cancer and dialysis clinics.[19]

A 2007 report by Public Citizen's Health Research Group found that about 60 percent of poor Americans are not covered by Medicaid.[20] That percentage is probably higher today. Those who are underinsured also have barriers in their way to care, especially if cost-sharing requirements of their plans are too burdensome.

Important as insurance is, however, whether one has coverage does not account for many health disparities. A recent study of more than 143,000 U.S. adults treated for cancer under traditional Medicare, without cost-sharing, between 1992 and 2002 found that:[21]

- Among people with early-stage lung cancer, African-Americans were 19 percent less likely to have tumors surgically removed than Caucasians.
- Among patients with colon cancer, African-Americans were 24 percent less likely to receive chemotherapy after surgery than Caucasians.
- Among those who had lumpectomy for breast cancer, African-American women were 7 percent less likely to get radiation therapy than Caucasian women.
- Among racial and ethnic minority groups, there can be other confounding variables that further challenge our capacity to deliver effective cancer care. Cultural beliefs and misconceptions account for some of them. As examples, one study of Hispanic women found pervasive fatalism that cancer cannot be cured and amounts to a death sentence,[22] while another study by the American Cancer Society reported that 41 percent of respondents, especially African-Americans, believe that cancer surgery can spread disease throughout the body.[23] For many Chinese, cancer is a stigma, which patients may try to keep secret, even from family members.[24]

In view of all these complexities, it comes as no surprise that researchers at the Yale Cancer Center, based on their study of racial disparities in cancer therapy between 1992 and 2002, concluded that: "[even among Medicare beneficiaries with cancer] Efforts in the last decade to mitigate cancer therapy disparities appear to have been unsuccessful."[25]

So we need to re-double our efforts to decrease these disparities within a coherent strategy to reform health care financing and delivery of care.

### 3. Over-emphasis on treatment can limit the continuum of cancer care.

The predominant focus of much of cancer care in this country is on treatment, with less priority given to other important aspects along the continuum of cancer care. Increased priority and effort needs to be directed to prevention and screening, as well as to improved care of cancer survivors and palliative care.

Cessation of smoking and other uses of tobacco products could make the single biggest impact on reducing the prevalence of cancer. According to the American Cancer Society, smoking accounts for at least 30 percent of all cancer deaths and is associated with increased risk of at least 15 types of cancer.[26] Yet efforts to deal with this public health threat have fallen far short of the mark. While the tobacco industry postures at social responsibility in its advertising campaign against teenage smoking, it battles against regulation of its products by the FDA. In 2003, the industry budget for advertising and promotion outspent the combined spending on cancer care by drug companies, philanthropies, and the federal government.[27] In 2005, tobacco companies spent more than $1 million a day sponsoring events and giveaways aimed to increase smoking among college students.[28]

Prevention of cancer in high-risk people can also be effective, but these approaches are likely to involve significant expense and disparities of access (e.g., for drugs such as tamoxifen or Evista (raloxifene) for post-menopausal women at high risk for breast cancer). Disparities in access, particularly for minorities, are complicated, based on such factors as distrust of the medical system, cultural beliefs, language and communication problems. But many experts believe that our lack of a national health care system is a major barrier to access to prevention and screening for cancer. Deborah Erwin, Director of the Office of Cancer Health Disparities at Roswell Park Cancer Institute in New York, puts it this way:

"Poverty and the lack of comprehensive health care are bigger issues than our communication problems, because you don't see these (health) disparities in Canada, where there is a very diverse population [and universal health care]."[29]

Farther along the continuum of cancer care, there are now an estimated 12 million cancer survivors in the country.[30] Six of ten survivors are over 65 years of age, most with one or more co-morbidities ranging from heart disease to diabetes, arthritis, and dementia.[31,32] Care has to be individualized for each survivor, taking into account a wide range of factors, including co-morbidities, health status, psychosocial issues, personal and family values, functional limitations, and quality (not just quantity) of life. The extent of survivor concerns is suggested by Figure 4.1, reflecting the leading cancer-related problems by time since diagnosis of cancer among more than 15,000 cancer survivors surveyed by the American Cancer Society.[33]

FIGURE 4.1

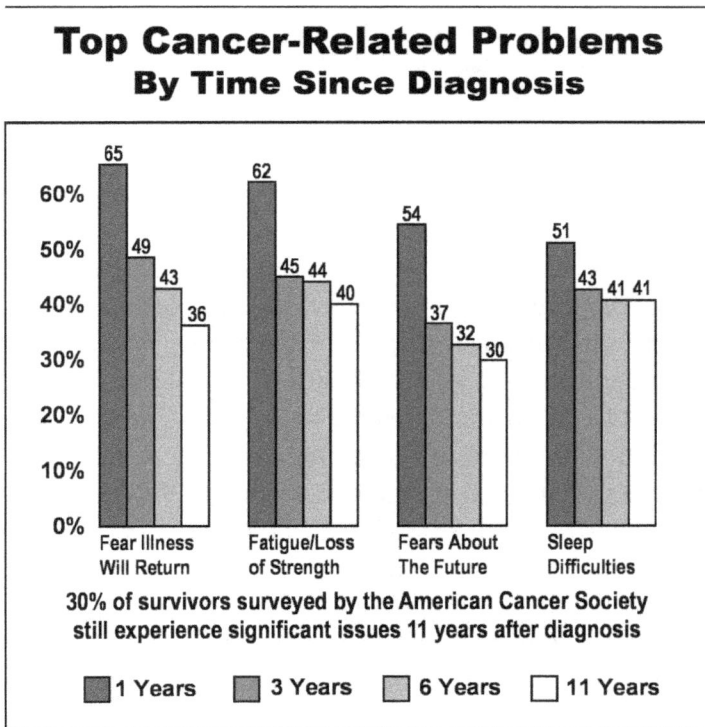

**Top Cancer-Related Problems By Time Since Diagnosis**

30% of survivors surveyed by the American Cancer Society still experience significant issues 11 years after diagnosis

Source: LaTour K. Healing well: challenges in cancer survivorship. *CURE*, Spring 2008.

Psychosocial issues pose major problems for most cancer patients, often under-recognized and inadequately treated. A just published book by the Institute of Medicine, *Cancer Care for the Whole Patient: Meeting Psychosocial Health Needs*, details the extent of this need. Nancy Adler, Ph.D., Professor of Medical Psychology at the University of California, San Francisco, has this to say:

> "Americans place a high premium on new technologies to solve our health care needs. However, technology alone is not enough. Health is determined not just by biological processes but by people's emotions, behaviors, and social relationships. Sadly, these factors are often ignored or not defined as part of health care. Many doubt their importance and dismiss the evidence as being based on "soft science." Even when acknowledged, they are often seen as ancillary rather than central to care. High and escalating health care costs fuel the argument that addressing such concerns is a luxury rather than a necessity. These views fly in the face of evidence of the important role that psychosocial factors play in disease onset and progression, not to mention their impact on people's ability to function and maintain a positive quality of life."[34]

Many cancer survivors develop depression, anxiety disorders, and even symptoms that meet the criteria for post-traumatic stress disorder (PTSD).[35,36] When untreated, these patients report lower social and overall functioning, and are more susceptible to sleep problems, fatigue, and pain.[37] Cancer survivors frequently have to cope with financial burdens and the emotional toll of long-term care, often with adverse side effects of their treatment. And of course, caregivers of cancer patients often themselves become depressed, and are at risk for other health problems and premature death. A 1999 study found that those reporting strain from providing supportive care to their spouse are 63 percent more likely to die within 4 years than are others their age.[38]

Another important part of cancer care, which until recently was largely neglected, is palliative care, focused directly on improving the quality of life of cancer patients and their families. Palliative care does not require that cancer patients give up on the possibilities of curative medicine, but does afford them a better chance to improve their quality of life over the course of their treatment, whatever their prognosis. Betty Ferrell, Ph.D., RN, nurse researcher at the City of Hope in California, has been a national leader in the development of palliative care as an essential part of cancer care across all phases of disease, whether initial diagnosis, treatment, remission, recurrence, long-term survivorship, or end-of-life care. As she points out:

> "The life-threatening nature of cancer – even in early stages and despite major treatment advances – is often met by denial and avoidance of the enormous physical, psychological, social, and spiritual consequences... not speaking of quality-of-life concerns doesn't make them go away. In fact, silence intensifies the suffering associated with unmet needs... Fortunately, since the 1990s, palliative care has become an essential aspect of cancer care. Palliative care 'upstreams' the great work of hospice and integrates excellent symptom control, psychosocial support, spiritual care, and other elements of whole-person care into the usual care of cancer, regardless of treatment or prognosis."[39]

In 2006, palliative medicine was recognized as a medical subspecialty by the American Board of Medical Specialties. Where available, palliative care teams treat common symptoms of cancer patients, including pain, fatigue, anxiety, shortness of breath, and depression. Care teams can include physicians, nurses, physical therapists, nutritionists, social workers and chaplains. Aside from medication, pain control may involve use of various kinds of nerve blocks and pain pumps, acupuncture, or transcutaneous electrical nerve stimulation (TENS).

A number of studies and reports have already demonstrated that palliative care can improve the quality of life of cancer patients.[40-44] But there is still a pressing need to expand the number of palliative care programs across the country in various treatment settings, whether affiliated with hospitals, outpatient clinics or other community-based programs.

## 4. Coordination and collaboration between primary care and oncology is often inadequate.

The broad scope of cancer care as just described is a big order, more than either oncologists or primary care physicians can do on their own. Close coordination and collaboration is an obvious requirement if this scope of care is to be available to all patients with cancer. For the best quality of care, both fields must be involved, working together to bring their own strengths to patient care.

Primary care physicians may, or may not, have been involved in cancer screening and the initial diagnosis of cancer. Whatever the case, when cancer is first diagnosed, they bring their knowledge of the patient, and hopefully of the family, to discussions of further management, as well as continuing to provide ongoing care of other medical problems. Oncologists and their teams bring their special expertise of treatment options over the course of cancer treatment and follow-up.

Unfortunately for many cancer patients, the care that they receive from their oncologists and primary care physicians is not coordinated. Whether followed primarily by either group, their care comes up short. One study of almost 15,000 five-year survivors of colorectal cancer, for example, found that patients followed only by oncologists were less likely to receive influenza vaccination, cervical screening, and bone densitrometry, whereas patients followed only by primary care physicians reported less screening by colonoscopy and mammography. Patients received the best care when followed by both specialties. Coordination really matters.[45]

Wider use of electronic medical records, of course, can facilitate better communication and coordination of care by oncologists and primary care physicians. But we need to rebuild a declining primary care workforce, and their respective roles need to be discussed, clarified, and individualized in each case.

## 5. Patients need to be more involved in shared clinical decision-making.

Medicine has a long history of clinical decision-making being the main prerogative of the physician. But the paternalistic "doctor knows best" model of decision-making leaves out many important considerations. Patient preferences and values need to be integrated into clinical decisions, particularly when tradeoffs are involved, as they usually are in cancer care, between benefits and harms of screening and treatment. As cancer care has become more technologically sophisticated in recent decades, there is often no single best approach in individual cases, so that informed patient preferences are essential to choices among alternative approaches and outcomes.

With the advent of the Internet and the Information Age, patients have ready access to much more information, thereby removing much of the information asymmetry of the historic physician-patient relationship. But since patients with cancer face an often bewildering array of choices amidst uncertainty, more information can add to their confusion. Most patients want to be more involved in their own choices of care, but need support in doing so.[46,47]

There is growing evidence that the quality of decision-making based on standard counseling in clinical practice is inadequate.[48,49] Many patients do not receive cancer treatments or screening tests that they value.[50] And practitioners have biases based on their professional area of expertise. Patients often expect no bias, thinking that their doctor is an impartial scientist simply relaying the facts. Yet, patients seeing a urologist are likely to be advised to have surgical removal of the cancer, while those seeing radiation oncologists are usually advised to have radiotherapy.[51] Many physicians are slow to embrace shared decision-making with patients because of lack of time, little comfort or experience with that kind of decision-making, or lack of awareness of patient values and circumstances.[52]

High quality cancer care requires a new model of clinical decision-making, one that incorporates patient preferences through the active participation by patients with their physicians in making their individual choices of care. Table 4.1 lists some examples of preference-sensitive decisions that benefit from this approach.[53,54] As an example of the effectiveness of shared decision-making, women with breast cancer who are empowered by shared decision-making have been found to be more satisfied with their care, to have overall higher quality of life, physical and social functioning, and to report fewer side effects of treatment.[55,56]

The last decade has seen rapid development of a variety of decision aids to help patients sort through their options more effectively. International criteria have been developed by a group of experts from 14 countries to judge the quality of these decision aids (see Appendix).[57] Some of these aids can provide patients with risks and benefits of treatment choices specific to their age, type, stage and grade of cancer. Use of these decision aids can help to reduce overuse of some aggressive interventions, such as orchiectomy for prostate cancer, and

Table 4.1

# Examples of Preference-Sensitive Cancer Decisions

Tamoxifen for chemoprevention

Genetic testing

Prostate-specific antigen screening

Early-stage breast or prostate cancer treatment

When to stop active treatment

Location of care at end of life

Source: Stacey D, Samant R, Bennett C. Decision making in oncology: A review of patient decision aids to support patient participation. *CA Cancer J Clin* 58: 293-304, 2008.

increase use of useful approaches, such as screening for colon cancer. One study, for example, has shown that women with early-stage breast cancer who used a decision aid were more likely to choose lumpectomy instead of mastectomy.[58]

## 6. The scope of cancer research needs to be expanded.

Despite the well-deserved reputation of the National Cancer Institute for high quality research over many years, the amount and scope of research in this country is much too limited to inform many clinical questions which arise every day in practice. Only one to two percent of all eligible cancer patients are enrolled in clinical trials. Moreover, these trials tend not to focus on the elderly, who carry the largest burden of cancer. A 2007 article in the *Journal of Clinical Oncology noted*:

"The traditional way in which cancer is studied – by clinical trials focusing on younger, healthier patients – has left us devoid of useful data with which to treat older patients in an evidence-based fashion. Not only have these earlier trials failed to establish the relative efficacy of cancer treatment in the elderly, but they also were unable to provide information related to the short- and long-term complications of treatment including decline in function."[59]

In view of the skyrocketing costs of cancer drugs, Dr. Lee Newcomer, as an oncologist and health insurance executive, adds this observation:

"The cost of these drugs is going to force us to take a more disciplined approach. We should not necessarily be refusing to reimburse for the 'experimental' use of biologics, but we should be enrolling those patients into a clinical trial so that we can gather information quickly about what works and what doesn't. We subject thousands of cancer patients to toxic treatments that may or may not help them. While we are treating those patients, we are also failing to collect the data to determine if the particular drug is effective. We can't afford to waste resources like that."[60]

While rigorous randomized clinical trials remain the gold standard for answering many basic questions, they are ill-suited to inform many other practical questions about the diagnosis and treatment of cancer. Furthermore, most patients receiving one or another kind of treatment for cancer are not followed by cancer registries, and we have neither the infrastructure nor sufficient incentives to learn in an organized way from the experience of patients. As a result, for example, it took many years to learn that high-dose chemotherapy with autologous bone marrow or stem cell transplantation for metastatic breast cancer did not increase the survival of patients, while it subjected them to increased mortality from the procedure itself, toxicity of treatments, and limited quality of life. More recently, Avastin, widely heralded as a miracle drug, was given to many patients with pancreatic cancer, again with high cost and toxicity, until it became clear that the drug had no value for this cancer.

More than science, market forces drive the adoption and use of many new approaches to the diagnosis and treatment of cancer. There are many reasons for this state of affairs. We live in a culture where technology is worshipped and "new is better." The FDA's approval process is industry-friendly, and the agency is not permitted (by law!) from applying cost-effectiveness criteria in its review of applications. Industry-sponsored drug research may be biased in favor of their drugs, often omitting publication of negative results. Off-label use of drugs (without FDA approval for the indication of use) is widespread, serving the interests of drug manufacturers and patient advocacy groups. Moreover, it is very expensive in time and effort to develop a framework to monitor and collate the experience of patients with various treatment regimens, whether in academic or community settings. That it can be done, however, is shown by the experience of cancer research in Europe, where some studies even evaluate the outcomes over time of *non-treatment*.

There are some early indications that this situation may be starting to change. The Centers for Disease Control and Prevention (CDC) established a program in 1992 – the National Program of Cancer Registries-Cancer Surveillance System (NPCR-CSS). Since then, cancer registries have been started in almost all of the states and territories. Some patient advocacy organizations, heretofore promoting early use of "new" technologies no matter how experimental or without evidence of effectiveness, are now supporting a more deliberate, science-based approach. Some clinical trial research is being developed on regional levels, as illustrated by the Southern California Kaiser Permanente Oncology Research Program's recent trials, including 250 patients in trials of the use of raloxifene in high-risk women to prevent breast cancer and the use of bevacuzumab (Avastin) to extend the lives of patients with colon cancer.[61] Some insurers are also starting to become involved with how effective cancer treatments actually are. As an example, BlueCross BlueShield of Michigan, as the first insurer to pay for the costs of pulling charts and compiling information on treatment of 16,000 patients a year, is collaborating with the American Society of Clinical Oncology's (ASCO) national registry to collect information related to chemotherapy-related side effects and pain management, becoming part of ASCO's national study of some 25,000 cancer professionals at about 385 oncology practices around the country.[62] But we are only at the beginning of creating a more deliberate measured process that should have been put in place years ago.

## What Next?

As is clear from the foregoing, the present cancer care system leaves much to be desired. Despite our huge financial investment in cancer care, there is enormous waste of resources on unnecessary and even harmful care while leaving out essential care for many Americans with cancer. Our present system is primarily market-based rather than needs-based. Before considering ways to correct these inequities in the last chapters, we need to ask: what are the consequences of not getting needed care? In the next chapter, we find some important answers.

# References:

1. Cullen KJ. Sky-high costs for new drugs: Weighing enormous expenses against tiny extensions of life. Oncology Today. June 10, 2006: p 40.
2. Meyskens FL. Sky-high costs of new drugs: Weighing enormous expenses against tiny extensions of life. Oncology Today. June 10, 2006: p 40.
3. Hewitt M, Greenfield S, Stovall E, eds. From Cancer Patient to Cancer Survivor: Lost in Transition. Washington, D.C.: 2006, p 27.
4. Ries L, Melbert D, Krapcho A, et al. SEER cancer statistics review, 1975-2004. Bethesda, MD: National Cancer Institute, 2007.
5. Jemel A, Siegel R, Ward E, et al. Cancer Statistics, 2008. CA Cancer J Clin 58 (2): 71-96, 2008.
6. Kennedy BJ. Aging and cancer. J Clin Oncol 6: 1903-11, 1988.
7. NRMP. More U.S. medical school seniors to train as family medicine residents. National Resident Matching Program. Washington, D.C. March 18, 2010.
8. Hauer, KE, Durning, SJ, Kernan, WN, Fagan, MJ, Mintz, M et al. Factors associated with medical students' career choices regarding internal medicine. JAMA 300 (10): 1154-64, 2008.
9. Rosenblatt RA, Hart LG, Baldwin LM, et al. The generalist role of specialty physicians: Is there a hidden system of primary care? JAMA 279: 1364-70, 1998.
10. U.S. Department of Health and Human Services, Agency for Healthcare Research and Quality Web site. FY 2004: Research on Health Care Costs, Quality and Outcomes. Washington, D.C.: U.S. Department of Health and H man Services. Available at http://www.ahcpr.gov/About/cj2004/hcqo04e.htm.
11. Ahmedin J, Tiwari RC, Murray T, et al. Cancer Statistics, 2004. CA Cancer J Clin (serial online). 2004; 4: 8-29. Available at: http://caonline.amcancersoc.org/cgi/reprint/54/1/8.
12. Ibid # 11.
13. U.S. DHHS Agency for Healthcare Research and Quality: Program Brief: Health Care for Minority Women (AHRQ Publication No. 03-P020). Washington, D.C.: U S Department of Health and Human Services, May 2002. Available at: www.ahrq.gov/research/minority.htm#BreastandCervical.
14. DeLancey JOL, Thun MJ, Jemal A, et al. Recent trends in black-white disparities in cancer mortality. Cancer Epidemiology Biomarkers & Prevention 17: 2908-12, November 1, 2008.
15. U.S. Department of Health and Human Services. The Initiative to Eliminate Racial and Ethnic Disparities in Health. HHS Fact Sheet: Minority Health Disparities at a Glance. Washington, D.C.: U.S. Department of Health and Human Services, 2004. Available at: http://www.omhrc.gov/health.disparities/glance.htm.

16. Intercultural Cancer Council. Cancer Fact Sheet: American Indians/Alaska Natives & Cancer. Houston, TX: Intercultural Cancer Council, 2004. Available at: http://iccnetwork.org/cancerfacts/cfs2.htm.

17. World Health Organization. Closing the Gap in a Generation: Health Equity through Action on the Social Determinants of Health. August 28, 2008.

18. Ibid # 3, p 11.

19. Sack K, Zezima G. Growing need for Medicaid burdens states. New York Times, January 22, 2009: A1.

20. Public Citizen. Unsettling scores: A ranking of State Medicaid programs. Health Letter 23 (4): April, 2007.

21. Gross CP, Smith BD, Wolf E, et al. Racial disparities in cancer therapy: Did the gap narrow between 1992 and 2002? Cancer 112 (4): 900-8, 2008.

22. Frank-Stromborg M, Wassner LJ, Nelson M, et al. A study of rural Latino women seeking cancer-detection examinations. J Cancer Educ 13: 231-41, 1998.

23. Gansler T, Jenley SJ, Stein K, et al. Socioeconomic determinants of cancer treatment health literacy. Cancer 104: 653-60, 2005.

24. Lagnado L. In some cultures, cancer stirs shame. Wall Street Journal, October 4, 2008, A1.

25. Ibid # 21.

26. Seffrin JR. Ten years after tobacco master settlement agreement, much work to be done to combat tobacco use. Atlanta, GA. American Cancer Society. November 23, 2008.

27. Vanchieri C. National Cancer Act: A look back and forward. J Natl Cancer Inst 99 (5):344, 2007.

28. Wolfe SM. Outrage of the Month. Big tobacco targets college students. Public Citizen Research Group. Health Letter 24 (10): 11-2, October, 2008.

29. Covallo J. Are minorities benefiting from prevention priority? CURE, Spring 2008, p 32.

30. LaTour K. Healing well: challenges in cancer survivorship. CURE, Spring 2008.

31. Aziz NM. Cancer survivorship research: state of knowledge, challenges and opportunities. Acta Oncol. 46 (4): 417-32, 2007.

32. Bellizzi KM, Rowland JH. Role of co-morbidity, symptoms and age in the health of older survivors following treatment for cancer. Aging Health 3: 625-35, 2007.

33. Ibid # 30.

34. Adler NE, Page AEK, eds. Institute of Medicine. Cancer Care for the Whole Patient: Meeting Psychosocial Needs. Washington, DC: The National Academies Press, 2008. p xi.

35. Hegel MT, Moore CP, Collins ED, et al. Distress, psychiatric syndromes, and impairment of function in women with newly diagnosed breast cancer. Cancer 107 (12): 2924-31, 2006.

36. Bruce MA. systematic and conceptual review of posttraumatic stress in childhood cancer survivors and their parents. Clin Psychol Rev 26 (3):233-56, 2006

37. News & Views. CA Institute of Medicine's 10-point plan for more comprehensive cancer care. CA Cancer J Clin 58 (2): 67, 2008.

38. Schultz R, Beach SR. Caregiving as a risk factor for mortality: The caregiver

health effects study. JAMA 282 (23): 2215-19, 1999.

39. Ferrell B. Another deafening silence: Patients should demand palliative care, no matter the stage of disease. CURE 7 (1): 80, Spring, 2008.

40. Kenen J. The new specialty in cancer care: Palliative care is catching on in centers across the country improving quality of life for patients along the way. CURE 7 (1): 51-9, Spring, 2008.

41. Ferrell B, Grant M, Padilla G, et al. The experience of pain and perceptions of quality of life: Validation of a conceptual model. Hospice J, 1991.

42. Ferrell B, Hassey Dow K, Leigh S, et al. Quality of life in long-term cancer survivors. Oncol Nurs Forum 22: 915-22, 1995.

43. Hearn J, Higgenson IJ. Do specialist palliative care teams improve outcomes for cancer patients? A systematic literature review. Palliat Med 12 (5): 317-32, 1998.

44. Foley KM. Improving palliative care for cancer: A national and international perspective. Conference Report from the 4th International Cervical Cancer Conference. Gynecol Oncol 99 (3) (Suppl 1): S213-14, December 2005.

45. Earle CC, Neville BA. Under use of necessary care among cancer survivors. Cancer 101 (8): 1712-19, 2004.

46. Davison BJ, Gleave ME, Goldenberg SL, et al. Assessing information and decision preferences of men with prostate cancer and their partners. Cancer Nurs 25: 42-9, 2002.

47. Degner E, Kristjanson LJ, Bowman D, et al. Information needs and decisional preferences in women with breast cancer. JAMA 277:1485-92, 1997.

48. Stevenson AA, Cox K, Britten N, et al. A systematic review of the research on communication between patients and health care professionals about medicines: the consequences for concordance. Health Expect 7: 235-45, 2004.

49. Loh A, Simon D, Hennig K, et al. The assessment of depressive patients' involvement in decision making in audio-taped primary care consultations. Patient Educ Couns 63: 314-18, 2006.

50. O'Connor AM, Bennett C, Stacey D, et al. Do patient decision aids meet effectiveness criteria of the international patient decision aid standards collaboration? A systematic review and meta-analysis. Med Decis Making 27: 554-74, 2007.

51. Towle A, Godolphin W. Framework for teaching and learning informed shared decision making. BMJ 319: 766-71, 1999.

52. Gravel K, Legare F, Graham ID. Barriers and facilitators to implementing shared decision-making in clinical practice: a systematic review of health professionals' perceptions. Implement Sci 1: 16, 2006.

53. Wennberg JE. Unwarranted variations in health care delivery: implications for academic medical centres. BMJ 325: 961-64, 2002.

54. Stacey D, Samant R, Bennett C. Decision making in oncology: A review of patient decision aids to support patient participation. CA Cancer J Clin 58: 293-304, 2008.

55. Hack TF, Degner LF, Watson P, et al. Do patients benefit from participating in medical decision making? Longitudinal follow-up of women with breast cancer. Psychooncology 15: 9-19, 2006.

56. Street RL, Voigt B. Patient participation in deciding breast cancer treatment and subsequent quality of life. Med Decis Making 17: 298-306, 1997.
57. Elwyn G, O'Connor A, Stacey D, et al. Developing a quality criteria framework for patient decision aids: online international Delphi consensus process. BMJ 333: 417, 2006.
58. Whelan T, Levine M, Willan A, et al. Effect of a decision aid on knowledge and treatment decision making for breast cancer surgery: a randomized trial. JAMA 292: 435-41, 2004.
59. Lichtman SM, Balducci L, Aapro M. Geriatric oncology: a field coming of age. J Clin Oncol 25 (14): 1821, 2007.
60. Culliton BJ. Interview. Insurers and 'targeted biologics' for cancer: A conversation with Lee N. Newcomer. Health Affairs 27 (1): w 41-w51, 2008.
61. Press Release: Southern California. Kaiser Permanente honored for improving cancer care through clinical research. May 29, 2008.
62. Rogers C. Blues, cancer group unite to improve care, cut costs. The Detroit News, August 8, 2008.

CHAPTER 5

# Lack of Access Harms and Kills

"Cancer care in the United States is among the most technically outstanding in the world. However, the U.S. healthcare system is at a crossroads as it struggles to provide care to all its citizens. Significant numbers of Americans are either underinsured or uninsured. This limits access to the complete range of cancer care services including and especially those directed at primary prevention. This unequal access amounts to a form of rationing... The U.S. population is the most culturally diverse in the developed world. The heterogeneity of the population increases the challenges to the health care system to provide excellent cancer care to all who need it."[1]

*—Laura A Siminoff, Ph.D.*
*and Lainie Friedman Ross, M.D., Ph.D.*
*Department of Bioethics, Case Western Reserve University*

The consequences for cancer patients of poor or nonexistent insurance are devastating. For all types of cancer, the uninsured are 1.6 times more likely to die within five years compared to cancer patients with insurance.[2] Correcting this with good access means three things: care must be timely, appropriate for the patient's needs, and ongoing without gaps. The most important aspect of access is the status of the patient's insurance coverage.[3]

This chapter looks at what happens when cancer patients don't have insurance, or when the coverage isn't working.

## Access and Outcomes of Cancer Care by Insurance Status

### Access to Physicians

For the many millions of Americans who have trouble paying for medical care, access to cancer care is a special problem. At the most basic level, they find it difficult to find a physician to see them. Many physicians do not accept new patients who are uninsured or unable to pay the full costs of care at the time of their visit. A 2007 national report found that 40 percent of physicians would not see such patients, that more than one-third would not see patients with capitated health insurance (HMOs), and that one-quarter of physicians would not see Medicaid patients.[4] (Figure 5.1) As discussed earlier, there is an increasingly critical shortage of primary care physicians (less than 30 percent

## FIGURE 5.1

### Percentage of Office-Based Physicians Not Accepting New Patients According to Method of Payment 2003 to 2004

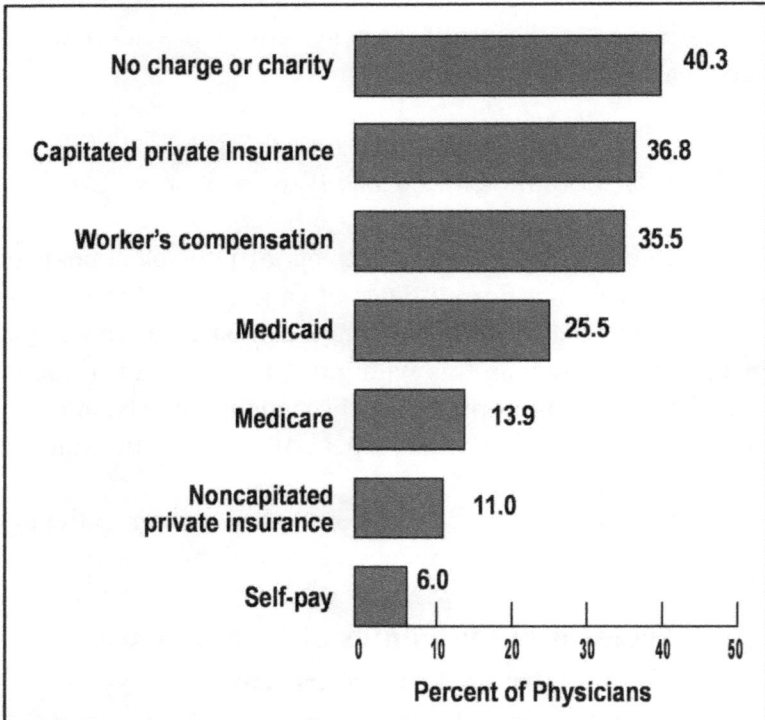

| Method of Payment | Percent |
|---|---|
| No charge or charity | 40.3 |
| Capitated private Insurance | 36.8 |
| Worker's compensation | 35.5 |
| Medicaid | 25.5 |
| Medicare | 13.9 |
| Noncapitated private insurance | 11.0 |
| Self-pay | 6.0 |

Percent of Physicians

Source: Hing E, Burt C. Characteristics of office-based physicians and their practices: United States, 2003-04, Series 12, No. 164. Hyattsville, MD: National Center for Health Statistics, 2007.

of U.S. physicians nationwide), so this problem is only getting worse. By 2011, only 42 percent of the nation's 354 million annual visits for acute care were to patients' primary care physicians, while 28 percent of these visits were to emergency rooms, 20 percent to specialists and 7 percent to hospital outpatient clinics, often with difficulty in arranging for follow-up care. [5]

While patients can be seen in Emergency Rooms for emergent problems, these services are very expensive, lacking in continuity or comprehensiveness of care, and it is often difficult to arrange follow-up care. A 2005 study, for example, found that patients with private insurance were twice as likely to receive a prompt follow-up appointment as were those with Medicaid, and that only one in four uninsured patients were offered appointments even if they agreed to pay $20 at the time of the visit.[6] Access to emergency rooms themselves is also getting worse as more safety net hospitals close their doors in counties with high poverty rates and as for-profit hospitals with low profitability leave their communities. [7]

According to a 2008 nationwide in-person survey of about 40,000 U.S. households (the National Health Interview Study, or NCHS), about 54 percent of uninsured people aged 18 to 64 years had no usual source of health care, compared to about 10 percent of people with private insurance or Medicaid. Among those uninsured for more than a year, 58.6 percent had no usual source of care.[8]

The primary care shortage is so severe that even seniors on Medicare have trouble getting access to care. In 2006, for example, only two-thirds of primary care physicians were accepting all Medicare patients who came to them for care.[9] Since reimbursement for many Medicare services does not cover the full costs of delivering services, it is likely that these numbers are even lower today.

A 2008 report by American Cancer Society researchers found that one in five of almost 8,000 older women with breast cancer delayed radiation therapy after surgery. Such delays have serious consequences. Women with Stage I breast cancer who delayed by 8 weeks or 12 weeks were 1.4 times or four times more likely to have a recurrence or a subsequent new breast tumor, respectively. Women who received less than 3 weeks of the typical 5 to 7 week course of radiation treatment had a 32 percent higher likelihood of death. Despite their coverage on Medicare, barriers to access included transportation, poverty, and availability of radiation oncologists.[10]*

**Cancer Screening**

A recent study by researchers at the American Cancer Society analyzed data for almost 600,000 cancer patients through the National Cancer Data Base (NCDB), which tracks about 70 percent of patients with cancer and collects data from some 1,500 U.S. hospitals. This

TABLE 5.1

## Cancer Screening by Health Insurance Status in Adults, 2005

| Proportion (%) | All | Private | Medicaid | Uninsured (at time of interview) | Uninsured for >12 Months |
|---|---|---|---|---|---|
| Women aged 40 to 64 years who had a mammogram in the past 2 years | 67.9 | 74.5 | 56.1 | 38.1 | 32.9 |
| Women aged 18 to 64 years who had a Pap test in the past 3 years | 83.6 | 87.9 | 82.5 | 68.0 | 62.7 |
| Adults aged 50 to 64 years who had a colorectal cancer screening test* | 44.2 | 48.3 | 39.6 | 18.8 | 14.9 |
| Men aged 50 to 64 years who had a prostate-specific antigen test in the past year | 33.5 | 37.1 | 20.8 | 14.0 | 11.5 |

*Had a fecal occult blood test in the past year or an endoscopy in the past 10 years.
Source: National Health Interview Survey Public Use Data File 2005, National Center for Health Statistics, Centers for Disease Control and Prevention, 2006.

Source: Ward E, Halpern M, Schrag N, et al. Association of insurance with cancer care utilization and outcomes. *CA Cancer J Clin* 58: 19-20, 2008.

study also included findings from the NCHS mentioned above. Concerning cancer screening, the researchers found marked differences in numbers of patients receiving screening tests by insurance status. Women aged 40 to 64, for example, were twice as likely to have a mammogram within the last two years compared to those without insurance. Table 5.1 shows the differences for four screening tests for patients with private insurance, on Medicaid, or uninsured.[11]

When patients are required to pay some of the costs for screening tests, rates of cancer screening drop. Among women in private Medicare managed care plans, those with cost-sharing get fewer biennial mammograms than those without cost-sharing.[12]

## Cancer Prevention

The uninsured are much more likely to have no regular source of care or health care visits over the last year than insured patients. They therefore have less opportunity to benefit from such effective preventive counseling services as smoking cessation, dietary and exercise counseling. A 2005 report, based on the 2000 NHIS survey, predictably found that patients without insurance or on Medicaid used less tobacco cessation aids than insured patients.[13]

## Late Diagnosis and Survival

The ACS National Cancer Data Base study described above, which found less cancer screening among the uninsured and Medicaid patients compared to the insured, not surprisingly also found that the uninsured and those on Medicaid have more advanced cancer when diagnosed. When treated, their survival is shorter. A majority of the uninsured had no regular source of care. One in four of the uninsured delayed care or did not get care because of cost. Figure 5.2 shows cancer survival by insurance status from this study.[14] The ACS researchers concluded that:

> "Individuals without private insurance are not receiving optimum care in terms of cancer screening or timely diagnosis and follow-up with health care providers. [Advanced-stage diagnosis] leads to increased morbidity, decreased quality of life and survival and often, increased costs."[15]

Also, as expected, more advanced cancer and shorter survival times are associated with both insurance status and ethnicity. For breast cancer, for example, insured Caucasian women had five-year survival rates of 89 percent, compared to 76 percent of Caucasian women with Medicaid or no insurance. For insured African-American women with breast cancer, 81 percent survived five years, compared to 65 percent on Medicaid and 63 percent of those without insurance. A similar pat-

FIGURE 5.2

# Cancer Survival By Insurance Status*

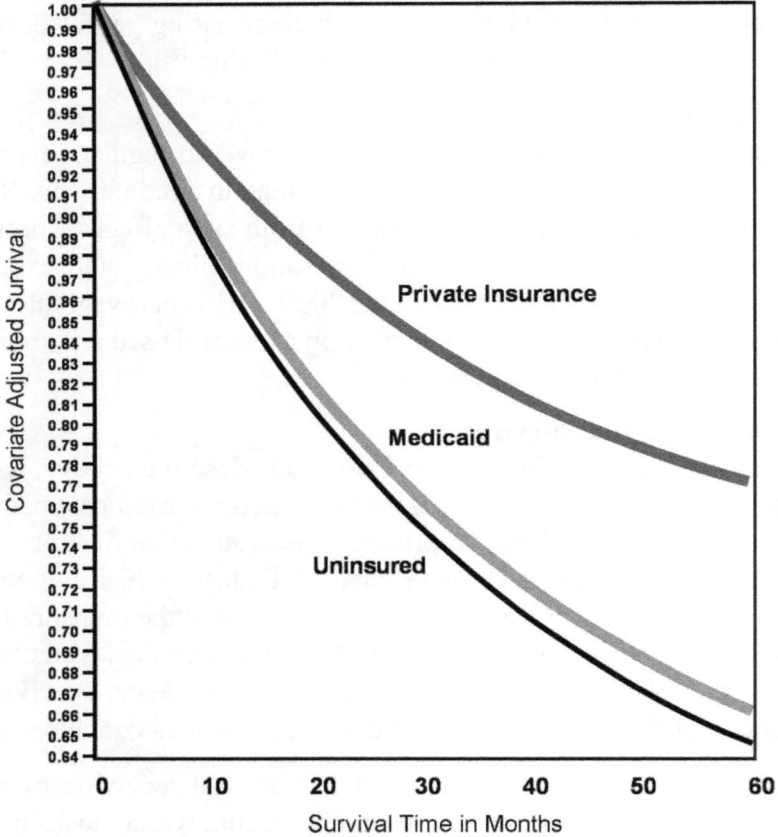

* Patients aged 18-64 years diagnosed from 1999 to 2000; excluded from the
analysis: unknown stage; race/ethnicity other than White, African-American, or
Hispanic; missing information on stage, age, race/ethnicity, or zip code. Covariates
included in the model are age, race, sex, and zip code-based income.
Data source: National Cancer Data Base
Source: Ward E, Halpern M, Schrag N, et al. Association of insurance with cancer
care utilization and outcomes. *CA Cancer J Clin* 58: 23, 2008.

tern, but with lower numbers, was found for colorectal cancer.[16]
**Survivor Care**

As we saw in the last chapter, for the estimated 12 million cancer survivors in the U.S., cancer is a chronic disease. Most have significant co-morbidities, such as heart disease, diabetes, and/or arthritis, and many have under-recognized and under-treated anxiety and depression. This vulnerable group of sick patients needs the best of survivor care, but here again, their insurance status is often a major obstacle to getting the help they need.

A recent national study examined patterns of care for more than 12,000 non-elderly (18 to 64) chronically ill patients in the U.S. After controlling for age, sex, race and ethnicity, uninsured cancer patients were three times more likely than their insured counterparts to have not seen a health professional in the last year (17.0 versus 5.4 percent), twice as likely to have no regular site of care (13.9 versus 7.4 percent), and five times as likely to use the emergency room for care (7.8 versus 1.4 percent).[17]

## Impacts on Families

The lack of health insurance obviously puts a much greater financial strain on cancer patients and their families than those with insurance. The 2006 National Survey of Households Affected by Cancer, jointly conducted by *USA Today*, the Kaiser Family Foundation, and the Harvard School of Public Health, identifies the kinds of stresses uninsured families have in dealing with cancer. Figure 5.3 shows a range of impacts confronting these families by insurance status. Almost one-half of uninsured families used up most or all of their savings, while 41 percent were unable to pay for such basic necessities as food, heat, or housing, and 6 percent ended up having to declare bankruptcy. This survey also identified these problems among the families with insurance:[18]

- 23 percent said that their insurance paid less than expected for their medical bills.
- 22 percent used up most or all of their savings.
- 13 percent reported that their insurance refused to pay for care which they thought was covered.
- 10 percent reached limits of what insurance would pay.
- 8 percent were turned away or unable to get a specific treatment because of insurance issues.

FIGURE 5.3

# Consequences of Financial Costs of Cancer by Insurance Status

Percent who say each of the following happened to them/their family member as a result of the financial cost of dealing with cancer...

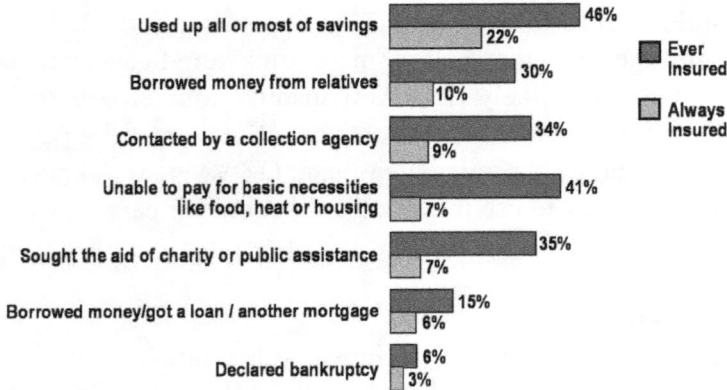

Source: USA Today. Kaiser Family Foundation/Harvard School of Public Health National Survey of Households Affected by Cancer (conducted Aug 1-Sept 14, 2006).
* Reprinted with permission from the Henry J. Kaiser Family Foundation. The Kaiser Family Foundation is a non-profit private operating foundation, based in Menlo Park, California, dedicated to producing and communicating the best possible information, research and analysis on health issues.

- 3 percent had to declare bankruptcy.

Here is one patient's experience that illustrates many of these problems.[19]

> *Dave, 62, is a retired landscape designer who had employer-sponsored health insurance when his wife was diagnosed with ovarian cancer. His insurance denied coverage based on the basis of her having cancer when he enrolled. The family was impoverished by the costs of her care, and she died. Dave now lives in a trailer on a friend's property, and recently paid off $273,000 in out-of-pocket costs for his wife's care.*
>
> *Now, himself recently diagnosed with neck cancer, hospitals are refusing hospital admission without $20,000 of his expected*

*$30,000 bill paid up front, which he is unable to pay. He has been rejected for "charity care" at other hospitals because he still has about $10,000 in a 401(k).*

Cancer patients on Medicaid or Medicare have their own problems in paying for care. Many low-income patients are unable to qualify for Medicaid (eligibility for a family of three in Missouri requires their annual income be no more than $3,504 a year!).[20] Cost-sharing on traditional Medicare can also be a major problem for cancer patients, as illustrated by this patient's experience.

*Robert, 81, a retired owner of car dealerships, thought he had good coverage through Medicare and an AARP supplemental plan. He has chronic myelogenous leukemia (CML) for which he takes Sprycel orally twice a day on a continuing basis. The drug costs $13,500 for a 90-day supply. His AARP supplement plan requires a co-pay of more than $4,000 for each 90 days. With his son, Robert Jr., they are trying to deal with the expense. As his son says "Somehow or other, myself and my family will do whatever it takes. You don't put your parent on a scale."[21]*

### In-Hospital Mortality

A recent study in California casts a bright light on how methods of payment for health care are associated with patient deaths during hospitalizations. Patients paying out-of-pocket were 80 percent more likely to die in the hospital (Odds Ratio = 1.8) (see Glossary) compared with privately insured patients; patients on Medicaid and Medicare had Odds Ratios of 1.6 and 1.1, respectively. That Medicare patients do so well in comparison with their younger and healthier privately insured counterparts is especially noteworthy since the Medicare age group includes higher numbers of sicker and disabled persons.[22]

## Being "Insured" May Not Help Much Either

The American Cancer Society study described above, as is the case with other studies of this kind assessing the differences between being insured and uninsured, may imply to many that being in the insured category gives good protection against the costs of one's future medical needs. But that is far from the case. There are many ways in which insurers can reduce or avoid their "medical losses", their term for payments for insureds' care. These include denial of coverage, cancellation of policies, and hiking premiums to unaffordable levels. As the cost of premiums continue to climb at rates four or five times those of overall inflation and workers' earnings,[23] the value of insurance coverage falls off markedly. Many insurers, both large and small, are exploiting lucrative new market niches for underinsurance policies of very limited value.

A 2009 report by the Kaiser Family Foundation and the American Cancer Society details the extent to which patients with cancer and other serious illnesses, even when insured, can be financially devastated by the costs of life-threatening illness. This report identified these five key gaps in our current system that put patients and their families in financial jeopardy, as well as force them to delay or forego life-saving treatments.[24]

"1. High cost-sharing, caps on benefits leave cancer patients vulnerable.
  2. Those with employer-sponsored coverage may not be protected from catastrophically high health care costs if they become too sick to work.
  3. Cancer patients and survivors are often unable to find adequate and affordable coverage in the individual market.
  4. High-risk insurance pools are not available to all cancer patients, and some find the premiums difficult to afford.
  5. Waiting periods, strict restrictions on eligibility, or delayed application for public programs can leave people who are too ill to work without an affordable insurance option."

As Drew Altman, Ph.D., President and CEO of Kaiser Family Foundation, concludes: "the insurance system often fails people when they need it most, when they get really sick."[25]

These examples show how limited many health insurance policies have become as benefits are cut back in order to attract purchasers and allow insurers to keep their medical loss ratios below 80 percent if possible (i.e., at least 20 percent for overhead and profits).

- Limited benefit policies, while much easier to afford, give new meaning to the word "limited" (e.g., policies with annual caps as low as $1,000 to $2,500, which in some cases cost more in premiums than actual benefits).[26]

- Insurers often add new restrictions in fine print, such as steep surcharges for top-tier hospitals and new co-payments for such services as cancer radiation treatments, which may render continued coverage unaffordable.[27]
- Allstate sells a basic cancer policy which pays a one-time benefit of only $2,000 if diagnosed for the first time with cancer (other than skin cancer).[28]
- Even a Blue Cross "catastrophic" plan cannot be counted on, as this patient found out.[29]

*Susan, 59, a divorced, self-employed artist and grant writer, purchased an Anthem Blue Cross plan in 2002 when she was in excellent health. She understood that the plan was not comprehensive, but figured that "at least I would be covered if, God forbid, I had an accident or got cancer. Two years later, when breast cancer was diagnosed, she discovered that her chemotherapy and other outpatient treatments were not covered. She is now $40,000 in credit-card debt, with premiums and out-of-pocket expenses consuming almost one-half of her income.*

Lest we think that a public safety net will shore up those unfortunate enough to be uninsured with cancer, this patient's experience gives cause for concern, even with a high lifetime cap.

*Jeanne, 53, is a free-lance writer on Social Security disability, Medicare and a Medigap plan (after a two-year waiting period); she had previous coverage under WSHIP (Washington State's Health Insurance Risk Pool for those denied insurance). She has been battling breast cancer for more than ten years. In 2006, when she came within a few months of breaking through the lifetime cap of $1 million under WSHIP, chemotherapy with Herceptin and Avastin alone cost $300,000. She joined an activist group that successfully lobbied the State Legislature to raise that lid to $2 million.*

*Jeanne is now on Tykerb, which costs about $3,500 a month. Her monthly income from disability is about $900 a month after* *health insurance premiums are deducted, but her co-payment for Tykerb is $1,600 a month. She applied to TykerbCare for a waiver of this cost, but was turned down since she has prescription drug coverage under Medicare. Worried about future costs, she is borrowing against equity in her house, and hopes that she can put off selling it for at least another year. Ironically but not surprisingly, benefits under Medicare and WSHIP are hardly logical or coordinated in the patient's interest. If Jeanne were to go back on Herceptin (given intravenously), Medicare and her supplemental policy would cover almost all of its cost, whereas if she were still on WSHIP, Tykerb would be completely covered!"* [30]

## Closing Comment

We have seen many examples of how our disjointed system of financing health care creates barriers to care, especially harmful to patients unfortunate enough to get cancer. The level of insurance coverage is a major determinant of the outcomes of cancer care. In view of the serious and increasing deficiencies of our current multi-payer private/public financing system, we will ask in later chapters whether we should replace it with a single-payer financing system, Medicare for All, coupled with a private delivery system.

Our present system, which gives care to those who can afford it and denies it to many who need it most, guarantees defeat in the war against cancer. That holds true regardless of what miracle cures are developed. Despite these system problems, however, many Americans either assume, or believe, that we have the best cancer care in the world. In the next chapter, we will ask how much truth there is to that view.

## References:

1.   Siminoff LA, Ross L. Access and equity to cancer care in the USA: a review and assessment. *Postgrad Med J* 81: 674, 2005.
2.   Ward E, Halpern M, Schrag N, et al. Association of insurance with cancer care utilization and outcomes. *CA Cancer J Clin* 58: 19-20, 2008.
3.   Ibid # 1.

4. Hing E, Burt C. Characteristics of office-based physicians and their practices: United States, 2003-04, Series 12, No. 164. Hyattsville, MD: National Center for Health Statistics, 2007.

5. Pitts, SR, Carrier, ER, Rich, EC, Kellerman, AL. Where Americans get acute care: Increasingly, it's not at their doctor's office. *Health Affairs* 29 (5): 1620-28, 2010.

6. Asplin BR, Rhodes KV, Levy H, et al. Insurance status and access to urgent ambulatory care follow-up appointments. *JAMA* 294 (10): 1248-54, 2005. 7. Hsia, RY, Kellermann, AL, Shen,YC. Factors associated with closures of emergency departments in the United States. *JAMA* 305 (19): 1978-85, 2011.

7. Hsia, RY, Kellerman, AL, Shen, YC. Factors associated with closures of emergency departments in the United States. *JAMA* 305 (19): 1978-85, 2011.

8. Ibid # 2.

9. Cunningham PJ, Staiti A, Ginsburg PB. Physician acceptance of new Medicare patients stabilizes in 2004-05. Washington, DC. Center for Studying Health System Change. Tracking Report No. 12, January, 2006.

10. Gold HT, Do HT, Dick AW. Correlates and effect of suboptimal radiotherapy in women with ductal carcinoma in situ or early invasive breast cancer. *Cancer* 113 (11): 3108-15, 2008.

11. Ibid # 2.

12. Trivedi AN, Rakowski W, Ayanian MD. Effect of cost sharing on screening mammography in Medicare health plans. *N Engl J Med* 358 (4): 375-84, 2008.

13. Cokkinides VE, Ward E, Jemal A, et al. Under-use of smoking-cessation treatments: results from the National Health Interview Survey, 2000. *Am J Prev Med* 28: 119-22, 2005.

14. Ibid # 2, p 23.

15. Sack K. Study links diagnosis of cancer to insurance. *New York Times,* February 8, 2008: A10.

16. Ibid # 2.

17. Wilper AP, Woolhandler S, Lasser KE, et al. A national study of chronic disease prevalence and access to care in uninsured U.S. adults. *Ann Intern Med,*149:170-76, 2008.

18. USA Today. Kaiser Family Foundation/Harvard School of Public Health National Survey of Households Affected by Cancer (conducted Aug 1-Sept 14, 2006).

19. Kirchheimer S. Cash before care. *AARP Bulletin* 49 (6): 20, 2008.

20. Solomon D. Wrestling with Medicaid cuts. *Wall Street Journal,* February 16, 2006: A4.

21. Kolata G. Co-payments go way up for drugs with high costs. *New York Times,* April, 14, 2008: A1.

22. State of California. Office of Statewide Health Planning and Development (OSHPD). Mortality in California Hospitals, 2006. Sacramento, CA, November, 2008.

23. Claxton G, Gabel J, DeJulio B, et al. Employer Health Benefits 2007 Annual Survey. Menlo Park, CA: Kaiser Family Foundation and Health Research and Educational Trust, 2007.

24. Schwartz K, Claxton G, Martin M, Schmidt C. *Spending to Survive: Cancer Patients Confront Holes in the Health Insurance System*. Joint Report of the Kaiser Family Foundation and the American Cancer Society. KFF Report No. 7851, February, 2009.
25. Ibid #24, Press Release. February 5, 2009.
26. Appleby J. Is a little medical coverage that much better than none? *USA Today* June 6, 2007: 1A.
27. Court J. Insurance: you pay, they bait and switch. *Los Angeles Times*, May 8, 2002.
28. McQueen MP. The shifting calculus of workplace benefits. *Wall Street Journal,* January 16, 2007: D1.
29. Future health platforms. Ill and underinsured. *Consumer Reports,* November, 2008, p 22.
30. Basler B. Million-dollar medicines. *AARP Bulletin* 49 (8): 12-14, October, 2008.

CHAPTER 6

# Do We Have the Best Cancer Care in the World?

Previous chapters have described many serious problems with cancer care in this country. But can't we at least take solace from the fact that we have the best health care system in the world, as is so frequently claimed? After all, many cancer patients the world over come to our famous cancer centers.

This chapter will answer that question by: (1) examining the case that we have the world's best cancer care, and (2) offering evidence against this claim.

## We're Number One in Cancer Care: The Incontrovertible Truth?

As we recall from Chapter 1, the rate of cancer diagnosed for both men and women declined by 0.8 percent each year between 1999 and 2005, together with a drop in the death rate from cancer by 1.8 percent a year between 2000 and 2005.[1] Moreover, consider these findings from various cross-national studies of cancer care in recent years:

- According to a major study reported in 2007 in *Lancet Oncology*, for all cancers, American women have a 63 percent chance of living at least five years after a cancer diagnosis, compared to 56 percent of European women; for American men, 66 percent can expect to live at least five years after diagnosis, compared to 47 percent of European men.[2]
- Compared to Canada, for all cancers between 2001 and 2003, five-year survival rates for American women were 61 percent compared to 58 percent for their Canadian counterparts; the same comparisons for American men were 57 percent versus 53 percent in Canada.[3]

- According to *Datamonitor*, an international market analysis company, 95 percent of American women are diagnosed early with breast cancer in Stages I or II, compared to 80 percent of European women; for Stage I colorectal cancer, five-year survival is 90 percent in the U.S. versus 80 percent in Germany and 70 percent in Britain.[4]
- According to the World Health Organization and the International Union Against Cancer, five-year survival rates for Americans with leukemia are almost 50 percent, compared to 35 percent in Europe.[5]
- A 2007 report of the Commonwealth Fund showed that 85 percent of American women between 25 and 64 years of age get regular Pap smears, compared to 58 percent in Britain; in that same age group, 84 percent of American women have regular mammograms versus only 63 percent in Britain.[6]
- Another 2007 report by Swedish researchers found that Americans have earlier access to cancer drugs than in many other countries; Erlotinib, a lung cancer drug, is 10 times more likely to be prescribed in the U.S. than in Europe.[7]

Based on all of those findings, how can we possibly not say that cancer care here is the best in the world?

## The Case Against the Claim that the U.S. is the Best in Cancer Care

It is true without doubt that some of the most advanced cancer treatments are developed here in the United States. But that isn't the measuring stick being used by proponents of the "we're number one" thesis. In claiming that survival rates for cancer are longer in the U.S., and using the data above, they are claiming that Americans receive better cancer care. The question is, are they right?

The five-year survival rates from the *Lancet Oncology* study were higher for all cancers in this country than those for 21 other countries studied (including some in Eastern and Southern Europe) – 66.3 percent for men and 62.9 percent for women in the U.S. compared to 47.3 percent for men and 55.8 percent for women in Europe.[8] Thus, it's entirely easy to conclude from these numbers that cancer care is better here than anywhere. Easy – and wrong.

When Americans think of Europe, we think vacation in a wealthy country, London, Paris, Frankfurt. So it's an imperceptible leap in logic to think that comparing cancer survival rates in the U.S. with those in Europe means comparing like with like. But there is an obvious error here: that would be comparing our country with a continent. Not a fair comparison, since Europe includes many poorer countries like Poland and Slovenia which have far more limited resources and access to care, thereby dragging down any measures that span Europe. But that's exactly what the *Lancet Oncology* study does. By using two large databases (US SEER and EUROCARE), it compares a country with a continent.

When European countries with more comparable resources are compared with the United States and the poorer countries are left out, wealthier countries in Europe fared well. In fact, five-year survival rates in such countries as Sweden and Switzerland were comparable to this country. Except for non-Hodgkin lymphoma, five-year survival rates of patients with hematological malignancies, such as leukemia, were comparable in US SEER and EUROCARE populations.

The *Lancet Oncology* study has other limitations when interpreted as McCaughey and the National Center for Policy Analysis do. These cross-national comparisons lack any information on clinical stage of cancers. This information is vital for cross-national comparisons because, to be meaningful, patient survival requires that patients be matched by stage of cancer. Survival rates of advanced Stage IV cancers will obviously be worse than lower-stage cancers. As the study investigators frankly acknowledge, a "major limitation of the EUROCARE data is the absence of information on clinical stage, which precludes comparisons of stage-matched patients."[9]

These stage comparisons really matter, and without them, the analysis is skewed and unreliable. Prostate cancer provides an illuminating example. The five-year survival rates for American men were 99.3 percent, compared to 77.5 percent for EUROCARE patients. But much of the difference between the U.S. and European five-year survival rates can be traced to the practice of more widespread screening in the U.S. Because we screen so much, we pick up more prostate cancers, most of which are early, Stage I, non-invasive, and slow-growing. When the investigators excluded prostate cancer from their statistical analysis, all of a sudden, the differences in the five-year survival rates for men with all cancers in the U.S. and Europe were cut by more than half. Because we screen more people for cancer in this country than in most parts of Europe, this same bias is likely a major source of error for other cancers in both men and women.[10]

In his excellent 1997 book, *Evidence-Based Health Care: How to Make Health Policy and Management Decisions*, Dr. J. A. Muir Gray, Director of Research and Development, National Health System Executive for Anglia and Oxford Region in the U.K., warns us about the hazards in extrapolating from comparisons from different databases, as was done in the *Lancet Oncology* study described above. He reminds us that *co-morbidity* is the presence of other conditions that may be relevant to a patient's outcome, and that *severity* describes the stage of disease a patient has. He further tells us that in comparative studies, these have to be accounted for. This was not done in the *Lancet Oncology* study. As he points out, this error is far from surprising: "Failure to correct for co-morbidity and/or disease severity is the most common reason why false conclusions are drawn from such databases."[11]

Actually, using five-year survival statistics for cross-national comparisons of cancer care is very unreliable and misleading, for several technical reasons well understood by health services researchers – *volunteer effect, lead-time bias*, and *length bias*. Behind those drab terms is an interesting story that shows what statistics can and cannot do, and how misleading they can be when pressed into service for an ideology like selling the U.S. health care system as the best in the world.

In their classic book *Clinical Epidemiology: A Basic Science for Clinical Medicine*, Drs. David Sackett, Brian Haynes, Gordon Guyatt, and Peter Tugwell, well-known Canadian physicians and health services researchers, tell us how earlier diagnosis of still asymptomatic disease through widespread screening will invariably render five-year survival rates unreliable and overstated for three reasons.

First, many studies have shown that people who volunteer for screening are healthier than those who do not volunteer. Thus the term, the "*volunteer effect.*" As one example, one study of more than 60,000 women randomly allocated women to two groups: one to receive no screening for breast cancer, the other to be invited to have annual mammography and clinical breast examination over a four-year period. In a striking example of this effect at work, the women who volunteered for screening did have a lower death rate from cancer, but also had only about one-half the mortality from heart disease and all other causes compared with those who refused screening. The volunteers for breast cancer screening fared better than the others even for diseases for which they were neither screened nor treated![12,13]

Second, when pre-clinical disease is detected early when still a-symptomatic, earlier diagnosis will always skew five-year survival to a larger value than is otherwise the case, through what researchers call a *"zero-time shift"* or *"lead-time bias"*. As a hypothetical example, let's assume that a group of cancer patients has a five-year survival rate of 50 percent from the time of initial diagnosis, with 10 percent dying each year over five years of follow-up and leaving 50 percent surviving at the end of five years. If we used a screening test that could detect their cancers one year earlier, when they were still asymptomatic, this group would have one more year of life (and one more year of disease) than they would without screening. This is known as a zero-time shift, which gives in this example a 10 percent improvement in the five-year survival rate. This "improvement" would hold even though therapy would not have taken place during that initial year or even if therapy is worthless.[14]

The third reason that five-year survival rates are unreliable is because screening more readily detects slower-growing cancers compared to faster-growing cancers. This distorts comparisons between different types of cancers. Researchers call this *length bias*. Lung cancer, for example, tends to be fast-growing, making it much more difficult to detect early compared to such usually slow-growing cancers as those of the prostate. A 1989 study found that chest x-rays every 6 months for early detection of lung cancer failed to reduce mortality from this disease.[15] This is not surprising since fast-growing cancers tend to have short preclinical periods, when detection might be possible, and also have more rapid clinical courses and greater likelihood of earlier death than slow-growing cancers.

Dr. Sackett and his colleagues sum up the impact of these three factors this way: "Early diagnosis will always appear to improve survival, even when therapy is worthless. Accordingly, we must insist on evidence from proper randomized trials of early diagnostic maneuvers before we act."[16]

A 2007 report by a group of Canadian and American health services researchers analyzed comparative health outcomes in Canada and the United States. They carefully evaluated the quality of studies and their degree of validity. Studies were rated low quality if they failed to adjust for stage of cancer. They concluded that Canada seems to have superior outcomes for head and neck cancer, and possibly for low-income patients with various other cancers. They found that American women have higher rates for breast cancer screening, and appeared to have higher five-year survival rates for breast cancer. They noted, however, that all, or even most of that advantage "may be due to the length and lead-time biases inherent in observational studies of screening,"[17] exactly the biases described earlier.

Concerning these three sources of bias inherent in using cancer survival rates as measures of comparative quality of health care systems, Dr. Stephen Taplin, from his base at the National Cancer Institute, sums up the issues this way:

> "The easiest solution to avoiding all these biases is a well-conducted randomized trial to observe the mortality owing to all cancers in an entire population and compare it to a set of randomized controls. By observing cancer mortality in the entire population to whom the intervention was offered, self-selection bias is avoided. Measuring mortality rather than survival avoids lead-time bias. Monitoring the entire intervention population for cancer occurrence avoids length bias sampling, so that the mortality estimates reflect the impact of the full range of natural histories.
> Unfortunately, randomized trials are expensive and physicians and scientists must sometimes interpret other types of studies. In these instances the interpretations must take into account these common biases."[18]

In addition to the above three factors which skew comparisons between five-year cancer survival rates, there is still another factor that distorts their use as quality measures of cancer care. Some cancers may be detected, and then regress and disappear without any treatment at all! This factor also would obviously then give falsely high five-year survival rates. Here is one remarkable and mysterious example:

*Charles, 56, was found to have inoperable liver cancer in 2005. He was told to get his affairs in order and that he had 30 to 60 days to live. But without any treatment, his cancer spontaneously disappeared, and he remains asymptomatic more than three years later.*[19]

There are a few other cases of spontaneous remissions of cancer reported each year.[20]

Another example, very real but not yet understood: a November 2008 article in the *Archives of Internal Medicine* reported the results of a multi-year study of some 200,000 Norwegian women comparing rates of breast cancer. Researchers in Oslo and the Dartmouth Institute for Health Policy and Clinical Practice studied two groups of women: one group had three mammograms over six years, the other has just one. All the women were matched in age and reproductive history, so that cancer rates were expected to even out by the end of the study. Instead, the women having only one mammogram had a cancer detection rate 22 percent lower than the more frequently screened group. This result suggested that some cancers had disappeared before they could be detected![21] This is a fascinating and controversial subject, which is certain to attract much more research attention.

All these seemingly technical details have in fact exposed claims of U.S. supremacy in cancer care as meaningless. They also give us an important lesson for the future. When presented with comparative survival rates, we should suspend our natural inclination to conclude that a longer survival rate indicates a superior health care system. Other outcome measures, particularly for mortality and quality of life, are much better indicators of the quality of cancer care than easily skewed survival rates.

So what can we conclude at this point about the quality of our cancer care? By one measure, we far outshine every other country in the world: we spend the most money – the most money in absolute terms, the most money as a percentage of GDP, the most money per capita. But for high quality cancer care, we should be able to expect that care is effective, that it is appropriate to the clinical problem, and that it is neither overused nor underused. On all of these accounts, cancer care in this country leaves much to be desired, as we will discuss further in the next chapter.

# References:

1.  ACS News Center. Cancer death rates and incidence down, annual report shows. Atlanta, GA. American Cancer Society, November 25, 2008.
2.  Verdecchia A, Fransiso S, Brenner H, et al. Recent cancer survival in Europe: a 2000-02 period analysis of EUROCARE-4 data. *Lancet Oncology* 8: 784-96, 2007.
3.  O'Neill J, O'Neill DM. Health status, health care and inequality: Canada vs. the U.S. National Bureau of Economic Research, NBER Working Paper 13429, September 2007. Available at http://www.nber.org/papers/w13429.
4.  Woodman R. Breast cancer diagnosed late in Europe. Reuters Health, March 3, 2003.
5.  World Health Organization. Global Action Against Cancer. Geneva, Switzerland, 2003. Available at http://www.uicc.org/index.php?id=497.
6.  Davis K, Schoen C, Schoenbaum SC, et al. Mirror, mirror on the wall: An international update on the comparative performance of American health care. New York. Commonwealth Fund, May 2007. Available at http://www.commonwealthfund.org/publications/publicationsshow.htm?doc id=482678.
7.  Jonsson B, Wilking N. A global comparison regarding patient access to cancer drugs. *Ann Oncology* 18, supplement 3, June 2007.
8.  Ibid # 2.
9.  Ibid # 2, p 793.
10. Ibid #2.
11. Gray JAM. *Evidence-Based Health Care: How to Make Health Policy and Management Decisions.* New York. Churchill Livingstone, 1997, p 143.
12. Sackett DL, Haynes RB, Guyatt GH, et al. *Clinical Epidemiology: A Basic Science for Clinical Medicine.* Second Edition. Boston, MA. Little, Brown and Company, 1991, pp 159-63.
13. Shapiro S. Evidence of screening for breast cancer from a randomized clinical trial. *Cancer (Suppl)* 39:2772, 1977.
14. Ibid # 12, pp 160-1.
15. Eddy DM. Screening for lung cancer. *Ann Intern Med* 111:232, 1989.
16. Ibid # 12, p 163.
17. Guyatt G, Devereaux PJ, Lexchin J, et al. A systematic review of studies comparing health outcomes in Canada and the United States. *Open Medicine* 1 (1), 2007.
18. Taplin SH, Mandelson MT. Principles of cancer screening for clinicians. *Primary Care*, 19 (3); 530-1, 1992.
19. Langreth R. Cancer miracles. *Forbes Magazine*, March 2, 2009.
20. Ibid # 19.
21. Zahl PHH, Maehlen J, Welch HGG. The natural history of invasive breast cancers detected by screening mammography. *Arch Intern Med* 168 (21): 2311-16, 2008.

CHAPTER 7

# Major Challenges to Meet 21st Century Needs for Cancer Care

"The evidence is conclusive that our people do not yet receive all the benefits they could from modern medicine. For the rich and near-rich there is no real problem since they can command the very best science has to offer... Among the majority of the population, however, there are great islands of untreated or partially treated cases... Although it is a principle of far-reaching and, perhaps, of revolutionary significance, I think there are few who would deny that our ultimate objective should be to make these benefits available in full measure to all of the people."[1]

*—Ray Lyman Wilbur, M.D.*
*First Dean of Stanford Medical School and*
*President of Stanford University (1916 to 1943)*
*Chairman of the Committee on the Costs of Medical Care, 1932 Report*

"In academia, and in private practice, the psychology of both doctor and patient, our engrained American culture of individualism, and economic factors will continue to be the strongest influences on the cost of care. Unless industry, government, and a substantial segment of the public agree that cost containment and a more just distribution of medical care is critical for the economic health and the common good of the country, cost containment will continue to be optional and arbitrary. Inability to pay and restricted access will be the tools for controlling medical costs – blunt tools that ignore justice."[2]

*—Joseph V. Simone, M.D.*
*Clinical Director Emeritus of Huntsman Cancer Institute*
*University of Utah School of Medicine,*
*Former Chairman of the Institute of Medicine's National Cancer Policy Board*

The above perspectives, by two leading physicians some 75 years apart, show an overriding concern about whether and how the potential benefits of medical care can be made available to everyone. Dr. Wilbur was a giant of American medicine in the first half of the 20th Century. During the Great Depression, he was called upon by the Milbank Memorial Fund to chair the important Committee on the Costs of Medical Care as the nation grappled with how to provide care to a vulnerable population in a desperate time. And Dr. Simone, with his long experience in cancer practice and policy in more recent years, echoes the same concern about access and equity of medical care. Today, as we drop into a serious economic downturn of still unknown proportions, their words are equally applicable to our times.

This chapter will set the stage for what needs to be done to bring modern advances in cancer care to all Americans, regardless of their income, race, geographic location, or ethnicity. We have three goals here: (1) to outline five major challenges to building a system of care to meet the country's needs in the 21st century; (2) to summarize how the current economics of cancer care are unsustainable in the long run; and (3) to briefly comment on how we might better allocate our resources for cancer care.

## Major Challenges to Cancer Care

These five problems stand out as especially challenging to the future directions of cancer care in this country. Some aspects of these challenges have already been touched upon in earlier chapters. But in view of the complexity of the issues involved, some repetition helps us to re-focus through a wide-angle lens before we shift to how to deal with these problems in Part Two of this book.

### 1. Rising Costs Reduce Affordability and Access

The introduction of new technologies for diagnosis and treatment of cancer are driving costs upward at rates at least seven times higher than the cost-of-living or median family wages. Cancer costs are rising by at least 20 percent a year.[3] Chemotherapy drugs are leading the surge in these costs. Oncology drugs now account for more than 40 percent of Medicare drug spending.[4] Some cancer drugs cost more than $100,000 a year (Erbitux for colorectal cancer).[5]

These costs are putting essential cancer care beyond the reach of more Americans every day, even for those fortunate enough to be employed and have health insurance. This patient story is unfortunately all too common.

> *Kathleen, 50, has been devastated financially by two bouts with ovarian cancer. She had raised three children as a single mother. She has had good jobs, a nice house, a decent credit rating, and health insurance. But today she has been bankrupted by medical bills, joining one million other Americans bankrupted each year for the same reason. After two difficult journeys through chemotherapy for ovarian cancer, she has been in remission for the last two years. She is trying to pull her life back together, but still feels that "a little black cloud follows me around all the time." Because of limited funds, she is putting off costly care for dental problems resulting from the toxicity of her chemotherapy drugs.*[6]

On the supply side, manufacturers have wide latitude to set prices at what the market will bear. Drug makers have patents for new cancer drugs giving them near-monopoly price-setting for about 20 years.[7] One might think that these high prices would discourage demand, but such is not the case. A 2005 RAND report found that health care spending dropped by only 17 cents for every dollar increase in price, showing that there is very little elasticity in demand by price.[8] We can only expect that patients with cancer are even less influenced by price.

With no end in sight for these soaring costs of cancer care, many in the cancer community are expressing serious concerns about access and affordability of future cancer care. Drs. Neal Meropol and Kevin Schulman, based at the Fox Chase Cancer Center and The Center for Clinical and Genetic Economics at Duke University, respectively, had this to say in a 2007 article on the subject:

> "Up to this point, our economy has absorbed relatively comfortably the increasing spending on health care in general and cancer care in particular. However, the continued introduction of high-cost novel cancer therapeutics and diagnostics (and those in other areas of medicine), reflecting scientific progress

and reward for innovation, is likely to exert increasing financial pressure on patients, oncologists, payers, businesses, and society. Thus, we may expect an increasing threat to our ability to ensure access and provide high-quality care to all patients."[9]

Thomson Reuters, which provides news and business information, reported in October 2008 that one in eight patients with advanced cancer (one in four with annual incomes less than $40,000) are refusing recommended treatment because of cost.[10]

The pressing question, of course, is: How can cancer care be provided to all Americans who need it without putting them through the indignities and increased stress of personal bankruptcy?

## 2. Increasing health disparities

Increasing disparities in cancer care are raising growing concerns within the cancer community as many studies have shown that individuals from lower socioeconomic groups and specific racial/ethnic minorities have greater risk and worse cancer-related outcomes.[11] These disparities are multi-factorial, including economic, cultural, and social factors, which impact prevention, diagnosis, treatment, and outcomes of care.[12,13] As we would anticipate, the uninsured and underinsured, Medicaid enrollees, and racial/ethnic minorities are more likely to have late-stage cancers when diagnosed.[14]

As we have noted earlier, for example, African-Americans have lower five-year survival rates than whites for most cancers at each stage of diagnosis.[15] Compared to Caucasian men, African American men have a 25 percent higher incidence of cancer and a 43 percent higher rate for all sites of cancer.[16]

The lack of health insurance, of course, is a big factor in creating and perpetuating these disparities. Racial/ethnic minorities are more likely than whites to be uninsured. According to the U.S. Census Bureau, when 15.9 percent of the population was uninsured in 2005, the uninsured rate for whites was 11.3 percent compared to 19.6 percent for non-Hispanic blacks and 32.7 percent for Hispanics.[17] Those numbers are likely worse today.

## 3. Variable, and often poor quality of care

Although we spend more money on cancer care in this country than anywhere else in the world, we are not getting the return in value of outcomes for our entire population. We still act as if resources are unlimited, and they may be for more affluent people who can afford care. But we still have two big problems: *overuse* of many cancer care services of marginal value, and increasing *underuse* of essential care for a growing part of our population without affordable access to care. The many bad outcomes for patients that we have already seen in this book are not isolated events. They are the result of chronic and entrenched system problems.

Many diagnostic and therapeutic services offered to cancer patients are of limited value. Some are even harmful. These examples make the point.

- At least 30 million full-body CT scans are being done each year for screening purposes at a cost of $800 to $1,500 each, despite the lack of evidence for such screening and without approval by the FDA or the American College of Radiology. These procedures subject patients to significant risk of radiation exposure, and often lead to further tests and procedures without clinical benefit.[18-20]

- Over-screening, over-diagnosis, and over-treatment of prostate cancer, the second most common cancer among men, is widespread in this country. A 2009 report of a randomized 10-year trial of the effects of screening for prostate cancer among more than 76,000 American men found that screening does not lower the death rate from the disease.[21] Instead, screening leads to over-diagnosis and over-treatment, often with attendant risks and complications that would not have occurred without screening. Scientific evidence is still lacking for the long-term effectiveness of treatment in early prostate cancer (confined to the prostate), whether by surgery, radiation, or hormonal treatment. A large prospective randomized trial has compared surgery (radical prostatectomy) with watchful waiting (observation without treatment unless the cancer is found to progress). Over 23 years of follow-up, that study showed no improvement in mortality or metastasis for men older than 65 years of age who had surgery. But radical prostatectomy is still performed in 60 percent of American men less than 75 years of age, often resulting in bowel, urinary, and/or sexual dysfunction.[22,23] These are serious complications for men who might not have needed surgery in the first place.

- Two newer drugs, bevacizumab (Avastin) and cetuximab (Erbitux) are commonly used for patients with metastatic colorectal cancer; they carry considerable toxicity, and increase lifetime care costs by more than $160,000 for median survival gains of about 5 months.[24-26]

- Many cancer patients undergo repeated imaging procedures and treatments well into their last 3 to 6 months of their lives with little or no chance of improvement. Providers have financial incentives favoring treatment over supportive care. Dr. Peter Bach, oncologist at Sloan-Kettering Cancer Center and former senior advisor on health care quality and cancer policy at CMS, estimates that 30 to 40 percent of spending on cancer care is of marginal value, with much of that unsupported by evidence-based clinical guidelines.[27]

- The anti-anemia class of drugs is the single largest budget item for Medicare and private insurers. Epoetin alpha (Procrit) and darbepoetin alpha (Aranesp) are commonly used drugs against anemia induced by chemotherapy drugs. They are very expensive, and highly remunerative to prescribing oncologists in ways that we will describe in the next chapter. As a result, they have been overused. A 2008 study by UnitedHealth found that 30 percent of patients receiving these drugs were not anemic at all.[28]

Quality of care is multi-dimensional and more complex than it may at first appear. In 1996, the Institute of Medicine and the National Roundtable on Health Care Quality (which the IOM convened) defined quality of care as "the degree to which health services for individuals and populations increase the likelihood of desired health outcomes and are consistent with current professional knowledge."[29] Drs. Mark Schuster, Elizabeth McGlynn, and Robert Brook at RAND added this definition for quality of care in 1998: "Good quality means providing patients with appropriate services in a technically competent manner, with good communication, shared decision making, and cultural sensitivity."[30]

Quality of care goes beyond what individual patients need, and must also include whole populations. In a 2009 article on the subject, Drs. Frank Wharam and Daniel Sulmasy at Harvard Medical School and New York Medical College, respectively, point out that three key obligations are engendered by the central act of medical care:

> "(1) health systems ought to maximize efficiency before engaging in explicit rationing; (2) savings should be distributed broadly across the population to facilitate the achievement of patient health goals, perhaps reserving a portion as an incentive for those individuals achieving these efficiencies and distributions; and (3) systems ought to promote equitable resource allocation."[31]

As we look at these various requirements for quality of care as they relate to cancer care, we keep coming back to the American Cancer Society's 4 As – care that is *adequate, affordable, available,* and *administratively simple.*[32] And as we have seen in earlier chapters, we cannot conclude that care is of high quality if it is ineffective or inappropriate. If a man with prostate cancer, for example, is rendered incontinent or impotent as a result of unnecessary radical prostatectomy when watchful waiting would have been better care, he has not been well served. As Sophocles said many centuries ago, such care may be a "remedy too strong for the disease."

## 4. Aging and Co-Morbidities of the Population

The number of Americans 65 years of age and older has grown by almost 10 percent since 1995, is now 12.5 percent of the entire population, and is tracking toward becoming 20 percent by 2036.[33] It is well known that most new cancers and cancer deaths occur in people over 65 years of age.[34] Since older adults who get cancer are likely to have co-morbidities, especially heart disease, diabetes, arthritis, and/ or dementia, decisions about the extent of cancer care may become difficult for patients, their families, and their physicians. When it comes to screening for cancer, for example, consideration needs to be given to an individual's co-morbidities, health status, quality of life, and life expectancy.

A thoughtful set of general guidelines for cancer screening of older adults is proposed by Barbara Resnick and Sandra McLeskey of the University of Maryland School of Nursing. (Table 7.1)[35]

Treatment decisions for cancer in older patients, who may be frail or functionally limited by co-morbidities, can be difficult for all concerned. Treatment may also limit quality of life and yet offer very little

## TABLE 7.1

# General Guidelines for Cancer Screening Decisions in Older Adults

1. For patients who have a life expectancy of <10 y, the focus of care should be on managing conditions in which the treatment is likely to be of immediate benefit rather than on screening for asymptomatic disease.

2. Older patients with multiple medical problems, chronic pain, or dementia may find routine screening tests to be more stressful than younger patients. This potential increased burden needs to be considered in screening decisions.

3. Screening decisions for older adults should be individualized rather than set strictly by age. The expected benefit of the screening test should be considered against the risk for each patient. Factors to consider include the immediacy of the screening benefit, the patient's life expectancy, and the patient's preferences (or, as appropriate, those of the proxy).

4. Coverage for screening procedures should not restrict coverage for older adults on the basis of age alone.

5. For ethical reasons, futility of care should be considered when decisions on screening or cancer treatment are being determined.

6. Quality assessment and quality improvement systems that use rates of screening tests in defined subpopulations as a performance indicator should not include older individuals for whom screening is unlikely to be of benefit.

7. Older patients should have access to screening tests for prognostic information, to inform families, and for future healthcare planning if that is their wish.

8. Screening should not assume that the individual wants to undergo treatment, and options should be provided that include treatment risks and benefits, as well as the risks and benefits associated with no treatment.

Source: Resnick B, McLeskey SW. Cancer screening across the aging continuum. *Am J Manage Care* 14 (5): 274, 2008.

extension of life. As an example, an unfortunately common dilemma now being faced by patients with metastatic HER2-negative breast cancer is whether to take Avastin. The drug was recently granted accelerated approval by the FDA for that indication, despite a 5 to 4 negative vote by an FDA advisory panel that cited a lack of evidence that the drug prolongs survival.[36] Under those circumstances, decision-making should recognize that diagnostic and therapeutic interventions may be medically futile (i.e., now defined as a situation where there is no evidence that intervention will improve the patient's current or future condition).[37]

## 5. How, By and For Whom Should Cancer Policy Be Formulated?

As is obvious from the foregoing, spiraling costs of cancer care now threaten access to essential care for many Americans unlucky enough to get cancer. This is all taking place in a policy vacuum where the market sets "policy" by default. Cancer is big business, with powerful stakeholders in such industries as diagnostic equipment, drugs, medical devices, and radiation therapy. But the increasing disconnect between what is brought to market and what is affordable and clinically useful is not sustainable, and it is cruel to those who are excluded from the potential benefits of care.

The cancer care community is often more focused on survival outcomes of individual patients than on their quality of life over the course of treatment, pushed along as they are by pressure from patients, their families, market stakeholders, and advocacy groups. Longer-term survival is, of course, a critical indicator of the quality of care, as are morbidity and quality of life during and after treatment. But we also need to be focused on population disparities by income, race, and other measures. And if we are to extend the best possible cancer care to our entire population, we have to include cost-effectiveness as an essential criterion of high-quality care. That takes us to the use of quality-adjusted life years (QALYs) as a necessary guide to policy making.

So how can these issues be addressed? The U.S. has a poor record in setting health policy. Two examples make the point. The former Agency for Health Care Policy and Research (AHCPR) had its mission limited and budget cut by Congress during the 1990s after an intense lobbying campaign by industry. Spinal surgery providers and device manufacturers were upset by AHCPR's publishing guidelines that favored non-surgical approaches to back pain over spinal-fusion surgery. There was more than a name change of the agency. When it became the Agency for Healthcare Research and Quality (AHRQ), its former mission to develop health policy was eliminated.[38] A second example involves Medicare, the largest payer for cancer care. It is prevented by law from using cost-effectiveness as a criterion for coverage and reimbursement decisions. As a result, the ship of cancer care continues rudderless as problems of cost and benefit mount and as access to cancer care remains dependent on ability to pay, not medical need.

Dr. Scott Ramsey, from his base at the University of Washington's Center for Cost and Outcomes Research, asks a basic question – "are we willing to restrict access to marginally beneficial cancer therapies because they are too costly for what they do?" He recognizes that as a painful question, but that doing nothing confronts us with this future:

> "If we choose to do nothing, as seems likely today, we will continue to have distortion in our system: historical trends where health expenditure growth exceeds gross domestic product by two-to four-fold (likely more so for our cancer budget); distortion within the health care payer community as payers who feel compelled to cover all cancer therapies will in turn restrict access to effective care for highly morbid and mortal diseases that the public isn't as aware or afraid of as cancer; less insurance in general as employers choose less generous insurance plans or shed their insurance benefits altogether; and higher taxes. If we are adequately insured or independently wealthy, we continue to get access to everything, regardless of cost."[39]

This country still has no effective mechanism to set cancer policy for the benefit of society, not just for individuals who can afford to buy care of whatever value. Other countries have developed effective ways to make allocation decisions and health policy, as informed by best available clinical evidence (e.g., the National Institute for Health and Clinical Excellence (NICE) in the United Kingdom and the Common Drug Review in Canada)[40,41] As a rule of thumb, the British have established a normal threshold of acceptable cost-effectiveness between 20,000 and 30,000 pounds (about $40,000 to $60,000) per quality-adjusted life year (QALY).[42]

We have yet to come to grips with cost-benefit tradeoffs. A 2006 survey of U.S. oncologists found that four of five feel that patients should have access to effective care regardless of cost; their implied level for withholding care was $300,000 per QALY.[43] In this country we can spend $364,000 for an additional year of life for one patient with lung cancer using Avastin therapy.[44] Imagine how much could be gained from spending that money on better prevention and early detection programs improving the lives of many hundreds of thousands of other Americans.

# Hitting the Wall:
# The Unsustainable Economics of Cancer Care

In earlier chapters, we have seen the rapid pace whereby new technologies are brought to market, and how they drive costs of cancer care ever higher at rates far beyond cost-of-living and what patients and their families can afford. We are already hitting a brick wall of affordability, but these trends go on unchecked. The costs of cancer care keep rising exponentially. According to Wall Street analysts at Morgan Stanley, cancer drugs accounted for 22 percent of all U.S. drug spending in 2007, double that in 2002.[45] We need to ask such questions as "Where are the limits?" and "How and who can put on the brakes?"

Although high costs plague most aspects of cancer care, the cancer drug industry is the poster child for the unaffordability problem. As prices of these drugs go up, access to their potential benefits goes down, and more patients and their families struggle with their finances as much or even more than with their disease.

The backlash to the increasingly unaffordable costs of cancer care is still in its early stages in this country. As a classic battle between private market forces and the public interest, it can only heat up. The growing un-affordability of cancer care has already reached crisis proportions. Circling back to Dr. Wilbur's concerns during the Great Depression 75 years ago, the question remains: what are we going to do about it?

## Should We Change How We Ration Care?

As you see, we ration medical care in this country, even for such a serious disease as cancer, on the basis of ability to pay. Health care has become just another commodity on the open market. This market is the main way that we allocate resources in this country. Can we develop the political will to establish evidence-based policies that can make effective care available to all Americans?

Dr. Daniel Sulmasy, mentioned earlier, is a general internist, bioethicist and Franciscan Friar who also holds a Ph.D. in Philosophy from Georgetown University. Recognizing that we need to better allocate resources, he suggests a common sense approach to rationing in favor of the public good by involving large groups of people in the pool to be rationed (e.g, by state or nation). In his words:

"Individual oncologists should not make rationing decisions at the bedside, nor should they be manipulated by financial incentives. Society has too much at stake in the maintenance of trust between practitioners and patients. Neither market forces nor bureaucratic barriers seem capable of attaining a just distribution of resources. Society can only maintain respect for the priceless dignity of each individual patient, while acknowledging that resources are limited if health care rationing decisions are made through open, public, participatory processes that free oncologists to act as advocates for their patients within the limits set by these processes."[46]

Market advocates tell us a deregulated market can spur innovation, bring more efficiency, choice and value to health care services, and fix system problems of access and cost. As the nation finds its economy in the tank and cancer care increasingly beyond the reach of ordinary Americans, we turn to the next chapter to see what markets can do.

# References:

1.  Wilbur RL. Interim Report of the Committee on the Costs of Medical Care, The Economics of Public Health and Medical Care (1932), as cited in Simone, J V. Health care access, quality and economics in 1932: The eloquence of Ray Lyman Wilbur. *Oncology Times* February 10, 2006: p 6.
2.  Simone JV. Ethics & medical economics: rationing care. *Oncology Times*, March 25, 2007, p 2.
3.  Newcomer LN. Oncology's perfect storm: The next decade. *Am J Manag Care* 11 (no. 17, Sup), S507, December, 2005.
4.  Meropol NJ, Schulman KA. Cost of cancer care: Issues and implications. *J Clin Oncology* 25: 180-6, 2007.

5. Chase M. Cancer tab. Pricey drugs put squeeze on doctors. *Wall Street Journal*, July 8, 2008: A1.
6. Stuckey M. When staying alive means going bankrupt: Health insurance didn't keep cancer-stricken California woman solvent. *U.S. News*. MSNBC, August 15, 2007.
7. Ramsey SD. How should we pay the piper when he's calling the tune? On the long-term affordability of cancer care in the United States. *J Clin Oncology* 25 (2): 175-9, 2007.
8. Ringel J, Hosek S, Villaard B, et al. The Elasticity of Demand for Health Care: A Review of the Literature and its Application to the Military Health System, Santa Monica, CA: National Defense Research Institute and RAND Health, 2005.
9. Ibid # 4, p 185.
10. Szabo L. Study: Many cancer patients foregoing care because of cost. *USA Today*, October 13, 2008.
11. Ward E, Jemal A, Cokkinides V, et al. Cancer disparities by race/ethnicity and socioeconomic status. *CA Cancer J Clin* 54: 78-93, 2004.
12. Institute of Medicine: Unequal treatment: Confronting Racial and Ethnic Disparities in Health Care. Washington, DC: National Academies Press, 2002.
13. Edwards BK, Brown ML, Wingo PA, et al. Annual report to the nation on the status of cancer, 1975-2002, featuring population-based trends in cancer treatment. *J Natl Cancer Inst* 97: 1407-1427, 2005.
14. Halpern MT, Ward EM, Pavluck AL, et al. Association of insurance status and ethnicity with cancer stage at diagnosis for 12 cancer sites: A retrospective analysis. *Lancet Oncol* 9 (3): 222-31.
15. Brawley O. Some perspective on black-white cancer statistics. *CA Cancer J Clin* 52: 322-5, 2002.
16. Jemal A, Tiwari RC, Murray T, et al. Cancer statistics, 2004. *CA Cancer J Clin* 54: 30-40, 2004.
17. Income, poverty, and health insurance coverage in the United States: 2005. update. http://www.census.gov/prod/2006pubs/p60-231.pdf.
18. What's NEXT? Nationwide evaluation of x-ray trends: 2000 computed tomography. (CRCPD publication no. NEXT_2000CT-T) Conference on Radiation Control Program Directors, Department of Health and Human Services, 2006.
19. Pennachio DL. Full-body scans – or scams? *Medical Econ* August 9, 2002, 62-71.
20. Brenner DJ, Hall EJ. Computed tomography – An increasing source of radiation exposure. *N Engl J Med* 357: 2277-84, 2007.
21. Andriole GL, Grubb RL, Buys SS, et al. Mortality results from a randomized prostate-cancer screening trial. *New Engl J Med* online. March 18, 2009, Accessed at http://www.nejm.org.
22. Bill-Axelson A, Holmberg L, Ruutu M, et al. Radical prostatectomy versus watchful waiting in early prostate cancer: The Scandinavian Prostate Cancer Group-4 randomized trial. *J Natl Cancer Inst* 100 (16): 2008.
23. Wilt TJ. SPCG-4: A needed START to PIVOTAL Data to Promote and Protect Evidence-Based Prostate Care. *J Natl Cancer Inst* 100 (16): 1123-5, 2008

24. Kabbinavar F, Hurwitz HI, Fehrenbacher L, et al. Phase II, randomized trial comparing bevacizumab plus fluorouracil (FU/leucovorin (LV) with FU/LV alone in patients with metastatic colorectal cancer. *J Clin Oncol* 21: 60-5, 2003.

25. Cunningham D, Humblet Y, Siena S, et al. Cetuximab monotherapy and cetuximab plus irinotecan in irinotecan-refractory metastatic colorectal cancer. *N Engl J Med* 351: 337-45, 2004.

26. Hurwitz H, Fehrenbacher L, Novotny W, et al. Bevacizumab plus irinotecan, fluorouracil, and leucovorin for metastatic colorectal cancer *N Engl J Med* 350: 2335-42, 2004.

27. Bach P, as quoted in McNeil C. Sticker shock sharpens focus on biologics. News. *J Natl Cancer Inst* 99 (12): 911, 2007.

28. Culliton BJ. Interview: Insurers and 'targeted biologics' for cancer: A conversation with Lee N Newcomer. *Health Affairs Web Exclusive* 27 (1): W 41-W51, 2008.

29. Lohr KN, ed. Medicare: A Strategy for Quality Assurance. Washington, DC. National Academy Press, 1990.

30. Schuster M, McGlynn EA, Brook RH. How good is the quality of health care in the United States? *Milbank Q* 76 (4): 517-63, 1998.

31. Wharam JF, Sulmasy D. Improving the quality of health care: Who is responsible for what? *JAMA* 301 (2): 215, 2009.

32. American Cancer Society. Access to Health Care. We're taking action. Atlanta, GA. Web site accessed June 21, 2008.

33. Moffett S. Senior moment. Fast-aging Japan keeps its elders on the job longer. *Wall Street Journal On Line.* June 15, 2005: A1.

34. Yancil R, Riles LAG. Cancer in older persons: An international issue in an aging world. *Semin Oncol* 31 (2): 126-36, 2004.

35. Resnick B, McLeskey SW. Cancer screening across the aging continuum. *Am J Manage Care* 14 (5): 274, 2008.

36. Washington E. Drugs in the news. FDA gives Avastin the green light. *CURE* 7 (1): 77, Spring 2008.

37. Bernat JL. Medical futility: Definition, determination, and disputes in critical care. *Neurocrit Care* 2 (2): 198-2005, 2005.

38. Deyo RA, Psaty BM, Simon G, et al. The messenger under attack: Intimidation of researchers by special interest groups. *N Engl J Med* 336:1176, 1997

39. Ibid # 7, p 179.

40. Buxton MJ. Economic evaluation and decision making in the UK. *Pharmacoeconomics* 24: 1133-42, 2006.

41. Laupacis A. Economic evaluations in the Canadian common drug review. *Pharmacoeconomics* 24: 1157-62, 2006.

42. Drummond MF, Mason AR. European perspective on the costs and cost-effectiveness of cancer therapies. *J Clin Oncology* 25 (2):191-5, 2007.

43. Nadler E, Eckert B, Neumann PJ. Do oncologists believe new cancer drugs offer good value? *Oncologist* 11: 90-5, 2006.

44. Ibid # 28.

45. Waggoner J. Pop quiz! How well do you know your finances? *USA Today*, August 8, 2008: 3B.

46. Sulmasy DP. Cancer care, money, and the value of life: Whose justice? Which rationality? *J Clin Oncology*, 25: 217-22, 2007.

# PART TWO

# How Can We Wage a More Effective War on Cancer?

CHAPTER 8

# In Sickness and in Wealth: How Distorted Markets Build Wealth for the Few and Jeopardize Health for the Many

We hear an endless refrain in this country that free markets are the only way to achieve greater efficiency, more choice, value, and quality through competition in an open market. We are told that this approach best fits our American culture of individualism. This ideology is applied to health care by conservative policy makers, market stakeholders and their lobbyists without regard to the damage wrought by such policies. These same forces argue that private insurance can best match personal needs, and that "one size can't fit all". The extent of ideological blinders is illustrated by this recent statement by Rep. Paul Ryan (R-WI) on a *Health Affairs* blog that was accompanying a report by government analysts which projects that health care spending will grow by about 6.7 percent a year to a total of $4.3 trillion in 2017:

> "These are not signs that the health care market has failed. In fact – and it is crucial to understand this – they are the predictable results of vast distortions imposed on the market over decades. The government is the single greatest contributor to this problem... "[1,2]

We have seen a polarized debate over many years, still unresolved, over the role of markets in health care in this country. One side of the debate is well illustrated by Ryan's words above and by Newt Gingrich below, taken from his 2003 book *Saving Lives & Saving Money: Transforming Health and Healthcare*:

> "To design an affordable 21st Century System of Health and Healthcare, we have to reverse the financial incentives

and encourage people to take charge of their own health and healthcare. The system would center on the individual who could direct the system by emphasizing personal choice. That would make our healthcare industry dramatically more responsive to the market, encouraging it to become more competitive, flexible, and innovative. In every market sector, that process of individual choice has meant higher quality, greater efficiency, and lower costs. Lower costs could help people afford healthcare and health insurance, enabling us to get closer to full coverage for every American."[3]

But there is a strong counter-argument that markets don't work in health care the way their proponents claim. At the other end of the debate, Daniel Callahan, Ph.D. and Angela Wasunna, Ph.D., bioethicists based at the Hastings Center in Garrison, New York and authors of *Medicine and the Market: Equity v. Choice*, weigh in on the issue this way:

"There is a market solution, many would say: let the market have its sway, not only giving people more choice than they now have, but also forcing choice upon them. They will have to decide whether they are willing to pay the high cost of contemporary medicine and the increased cost of new technologies or do without; it will be up to them. This may appeal to some people, particularly the affluent (as with medical savings accounts), but when the pinch of high costs comes to the middle class and those otherwise well off, they are likely to balk. They are then likely to turn to government for relief, as is happening with pharmaceuticals in the United States. Even if, technically, many people can afford the drugs, that would only be possible by sacrificing other things in their lives that are of importance also; at some point, the tension would be intolerable, and choice would be a tyranny not a liberation."[4]

As you have already seen in earlier chapters, our deregulated health care marketplace wreaks havoc on many millions of our fellow Americans. The track record of free market theories in health care speak for themselves.

By this point, the scope of the storm that the cancer generation is confronted with is starkly clear. The persistent questions remain: Can we rebuild our system to bring modern advances in cancer care to all Americans, regardless of their income, ethnicity, or location? And if so, how? These are the questions that we will address in this and the chapters to follow.

This chapter has two goals: (1) to describe some of the many ways in which markets work *against* the interests of cancer patients and their families, and (2) to briefly compare concepts of market justice and social justice.

# How "Markets" Fail Cancer Patients

The common wisdom of most health economists, dating back to the 1960s, has been that free markets can, and should, work in health care. Despite the many signs of market failure around us, they continue to deny the limits of markets. But there have also been some economist voices in the wilderness with warnings about markets in health care. Kenneth Arrow's landmark paper in 1963, *Uncertainty and the Welfare Economics of Medical Care*, called attention to many of the reasons that markets don't work in medical care as they do in other sectors of the economy. He pointed out these differences: irregular and unpredictable demand, uncertainty of outcomes, inadequate information, erratic supply conditions, and the need for non-market interventions and control.[5,6] More recently, Robert Evans, Ph.D., the distinguished Canadian health economist, summed up the matter in this way:

> "There is in health care no 'private, competitive market' of the form described in the economics textbooks, anywhere in the world. There never has been, and inherent characteristics of health and health care make it impossible that there ever could be."[7]

Turning to cancer care, here are five big reasons why free markets work against the interests of patients and their families even as they enrich those on the supply side.

### 1. Consolidation Makes a Mockery of Competition

It is a fiction that there is real competition throughout the health care system. Instead, we see consolidation that limits competition among hospitals, other institutions, providers, and industries. These examples suggest how little real competition goes on in health care.

- The Community Tracking Study (CTS), a project of the Washington-based Center for Studying Health System Change, is a long-term longitudinal study of hospitals, health plans, physicians and other provider groups in 12 states. Begun in metropolitan areas, employers, physicians, and households are included in periodic surveys. The CTS has identified these four barriers to efficiency in the markets studied: (1) providers' market power; (2) absence of potentially efficient provider systems; (3) employers' inability to push the system toward more efficiency and quality; and (4) insufficient health plan competition.[8]

- Large investor-owned chains, whether involving hospitals, clinical laboratories, imaging centers, nursing homes, or medical suppliers, dominate the market in many parts of the country. In El Paso, Texas, for example, Tenet, the second largest hospital chain, controls about 80 percent of hospital beds.[9]

- A recent study by the American Medical Association found near-monopolies by private insurers in 95 percent of HMO/PPO markets in 43 states; in 56 percent of these markets, a single insurer controls more than one-half of the business in HMO/PPO underwriting. These developments have triggered antitrust concerns by the Department of Justice.[10]

- The Senate Judiciary Subcommittee held a hearing several years ago on consolidation within the health insurance industry. More than 400 mergers have taken place over the last 10 years, premiums have gone up by 129 percent in the last eight years, and consumers often have little or no choice between carriers. Concerned about these impacts on small business, the National Federation of Independent Business launched a campaign for reform.[11] Figure 8.1 shows the extent of consolidation by market share of the three largest commercial carriers.[12]

- When it becomes clear that consolidation stifles competition, an easy remedy to reach for is anti-trust regulation: break up the market into scrappy players who will compete and restore the virtues of the market. But not so fast. It is estimated that a market must have a population of at least 400,000 before there can be any real competition among facilities or providers.

FIGURE 8.1

# Health Insurance Oligopoly
## A Few Plans Dominate Most States

Number of States

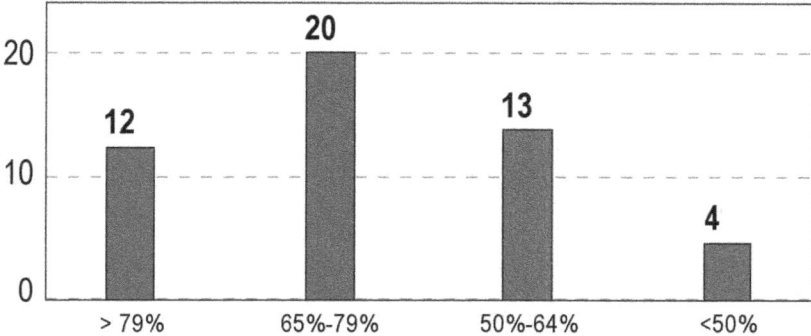

**Market Share of 3 Largest Commercial Insurers**

Source: Robinson, J C. Consolidation and the transformation of competition in health insurance. *Health Affairs*, November/December 2004; 23(6): 11-24

Anything less and the market is not big enough to sustain multiple competitors. The problem is that fully one-half of the American population live in those regions where competition cannot take place.[13]

## 2. Profits Trump Service

The business model, by which markets are necessarily structured, is designed for profits, not primarily service. Success is measured by market share, financial bottom lines, and return to investors. In the insurance industry, success is measured by medical-loss ratios (MLRs). Lower MLRs generate higher profits to the insurer by limiting payments for medical care. Angela Braly, CEO of Wellpoint, the nation's largest health insurer, is unambiguous on this matter: "We will not sacrifice profitability for membership." She further assures investors by saying that Wellpoint has the market power to "lean hard on its network doctors to accept lower reimbursement."[14]

The disconnect between the business model and the service model is consistent across the spectrum of medical care. Investor-owned care has been well documented over the years to be more expensive and of lower quality than not-for-profit care, whether by hospitals, HMOs, nursing homes, or mental health centers. (Table 8.1)[15-27] While market theorists argue that market competition will drive down costs, that is just not true in health care. Drs. David Himmelstein and Steffie Woolhandler, general internists and health policy experts at Harvard Medical School, explain why:

> "Investor-owned health care firms are not cost minimizers but profit maximizers. Strategies that bolster profitability often worsen efficiency. U.S. health firms have found that raising revenues by exploiting loopholes or lobbying politicians is more profitable than improving efficiency or quality."[28]

### TABLE 8.1

### Investor-owned care: Comparative examples versus not-for-profit care

| | |
|---|---|
| Hospitals | Costs 3 to 13 percent higher, with higher overhead, fewer nurses, and death rates 6 to 7 percent higher [15-21] |
| HMOs | Higher overhead (25 to 33 percent for some of the largest HMOs); worse scores on 14 of 14 quality indicators reported to National Committee for Quality Assurance[22-24] |
| Nursing Homes | Lower staffing levels and worse quality of care (30 percent committed violations that caused death or life-threatening harm to patients)[25] |
| Mental Health Centers | Medicare expelled 80 programs after investigations found that 91 percent of claims were fraudulent;[26] for-profit behavioral health companies impose restrictive barriers and limits to care (e.g., premature discharge from hospitals without adequate outpatient care)[27] |

Source: Geyman JP. *The Corrosion of Medicine: Can The Profession Reclaim Its Moral Legacy?* Monroe, ME: Common Courage Press, 2008, p37.

In essence, then, the ideological precepts of competition and efficiency serving the consumer in the health care arena are a fantasy that is precisely the opposite of reality: we have no true competition, we couldn't have it if we wanted it, and the mantra of efficiency as the road to profitability has been replaced by the easier route of loopholes and lobbyists.

It is not surprising, then, that in this "market" there are many examples of how the system works against the interests of cancer patients, from screening and prevention to treatment and survival care. Here are just a few of them.

### • *Gene Testing.*

A hot new market is opening up in the biotechnology industry for producers of genetic tests, so far with little oversight or quality control. California-based Navigenics and 23andMe are early leaders in the field. Genetic testing products are being marketed directly to consumers as "personal genetic information services," not medical testing or advice. Saliva samples are used for the tests. Genetic testing by 23andMe costs $1,000, while Navigenics testing costs $2,500. One company, Knome, is offering to do a complete sequence of a person's genome for $350,000. Critics point out that these tests may not be clinically valid, and that they are not backed by scientific studies. Perhaps just as important, having one's genome sequence may be a fun curiosity but is of little or no help in improving health because of this lack of utility. Regulators in New York and California have recently ordered these companies to cease and desist their direct marketing of these products to consumers.[29]

### • *Tobacco Industry Opposes Cancer Prevention*

The tobacco industry has never been a friend of cancer patients and their families, as it lobbies relentlessly for its increasing sales of known carcinogens. Recall from Chapter 2 that this one industry in 2003 spent more on advertising and promotion of its products than the combined total of funds spent on cancer by drug companies, philanthropies, and the federal government.

Long opposed to public health measures intended to decrease smoking and reduce cancer deaths, the industry struggles against declining sales of its products in the United States. It is estimated that cigarette smoking causes about 440,000 deaths a year in the U.S.[30] But the industry just gets more creative as it seeks to expand its markets. Philip Morris International (PMI) has recently been spun off by Philip Morris USA, thereby freeing PMI from regulatory, legal and public relations problems in this country.[31]

PMI recently made Robert Weissman's list of Top 10 Worst Corporations of 2008. As editor of the Washington, D.C.-based *Multinational Monitor*, Weissman describes PMI's goals in this way:

> "Philip Morris International has already signaled its initial plans to subvert the most important policies to reduce smoking and the toll from tobacco-related disease (now at 5 million lives a year). The company has announced plans to inflict on the world an array of new products, packages and marketing efforts. These are designed to undermine smoke-free workplace rules, defeat tobacco taxes, segment markets with specially flavored products, offer flavored cigarettes sure to appeal to youth and overcome marketing restrictions."[32]

As the leading international tobacco company, with 7 of the top 15 brands, PMI has more than 75,000 employees around the world.[33] Meanwhile, R. J. Reynolds has mounted a $25-to-$50 million dollar promotion campaign for its new female-friendly Camel No. 9 (in regular and menthol flavors), with such advertising slogans as "light and luscious" and with utter disregard for the fact that lung cancer is now the number one cancer among American women.[34] As pressure mounts in a number of states to enact increases in cigarette taxes, industry spends millions on lobbyists and campaign contributions in Washington as it also works in targeted congressional districts to stoke grassroots opposition to these tax increases. Paying no concern to the American Cancer Society's estimate that a 61 cent tax increase to a dollar a pack would prevent 900,000 deaths from tobacco-related causes,[35] industry efforts succeeded in defeating these added taxes in California, Missouri, and Oregon.[36]

- *Not-for-Profit Hospitals Forsake Their Service Mission for Profits*

So-called not-for-profit hospitals are expected to take on a service mission in underserved communities in exchange for tax-exempt status. But an increasing number of these hospitals are leaving communities of need and looking more like for-profit cash machines with creative and obscure accounting practices. Ascension Health is one such example. As the nation's largest not-for-profit system, it owns 67 hospitals in 20 states and the District of Columbia. With roots back to the Daughters of Charity in 17th century France, it is affiliated with the Roman Catholic Church and has a mission to serve all, "with special attention to those who are poor and vulnerable." But in Detroit, Michigan, Ascension's local subsidiary recently closed Riverview Hospital, the third hospital it has shut down in Detroit in the last 10 years and the only one remaining in the city's east side. Moving 30 miles to an affluent suburb, it is opening a new $224 million hospital. In the wake of its departure from Detroit's east side, many physicians have also left the area, including the only oncologist in the area. Riverside's Emergency Room has become an urgent care center, no longer required to treat all comers regardless of ability to pay, and patients are now charged $50 a visit.

The move paid off big for Ascension Health. Its net income almost tripled to $1.2 billion between 2004 and 2007, and its cash and investments exceeded $7 billion for the year ended June 30, 2008. Because of Ascension's tax exempt-status, each year taxpayers end up shouldering the burden caused by billions of dollars worth of Ascension's tax exemptions, giving new meaning to the term "nonprofit."[37]

This pattern of not-for-profit hospitals leaving urban underserved communities for more affluent suburbs is playing out all over the country, leaving behind hundreds of thousands of patients who are uninsured, on Medicaid or Medicare, and breaking up local systems of care. This trend is raising serious questions about the legitimacy of tax-exempt status for "not-for-profit" hospitals. They receive more than $12 billion a year in tax-exemptions, according to the CBO. Yet a February 2009 IRS report, based on a survey of 489 "non-profit" hospitals, found that these hospitals spent only 9 percent of their revenue on community benefit; more than 20 percent of the hospitals reported aggregate community benefit expenditures of less than 2 percent of total revenue.[38]

### • *Private Medicare Plans and the Part D Prescription Drug Benefit*

The Medicare Prescription Drug, Improvement, and Modernization Act of 2003 (MMA) is a classic example of the profit mission trumping service. Crafted by conservative legislators, K Street lobbyists and others with revolving door connections between industry and government, the MMA opened up lucrative new markets for the drug and insurance industries. The drug benefit was handed over to the private sector, and various types of private Medicare Advantage plans were established (PPOs, HMOs, and PFFS plans) (see Glossary). The MMA prohibited the government from using its bulk purchasing power to negotiate discounted drug prices, as the Veterans Administration does so effectively with discounts of more than 40 percent. Since most new cancers and cancer deaths occur in people 65 years of age and older, and since many younger cancer patients end up on Medicare after a two-year wait on Social Security disability, this legislation directly impacts the majority of people with cancer.

It was obvious from the beginning that plans created by the MMA would be less efficient, more expensive, and less reliable than traditional Medicare. This is exactly what has happened, as shown by these examples.

- Medicare patients today face a bewildering array of choices of plans for 2009 – almost 50 prescription drug plans and more than 40 private Medicare plans; information available to them from the companies or CMS is often confusing, incomplete, or inaccurate;[39] more than one-half of enrollees in private Medicare plans have no annual limits on their own out-of-pocket spending, and many plans exclude coverage for chemotherapy, as many patients find out the hard way.[40]
- Taxpayers subsidized private insurers by $8.5 billion in 2008, including payments by insurers to brokers, who received

$500 or more for each new Medicare Advantage enrollee in 2009, as well as five years of renewal commissions worth at least $250 a year.[41]

• Bait and switch tactics, predicted at the outset, have occurred; premiums for Humana's standard drug plan, the second largest in the country, have increased by 330 percent since its "low-premium" plan was launched in 2006; Humana has withdrawn completely from the low-income market for 2009, forcing many patients to change drug plans, and even perhaps also their physicians if the only cheaper plan for drug coverage is an HMO.[42]

• According to the Medicare Payment Advisory Commission (MedPAC), private Medicare Advantage plans cost the government 13 percent more per beneficiary on average than the regular Medicare plan in 2008.[43]

• The 10 largest drug plans increased their premiums for 2009 by an average of 30 percent or more; despite these premium hikes, 75 percent of drug plans and 56 percent of private Medicare plans offered no coverage in the "doughnut hole" gap ($2,920 to $6,596 in 2009) (see also Glossary).[44] Since most cancer patients have very expensive medications, most will get to know this coverage gap all too well, which has been a big present to the drug industry. In 2009, for example, most commonly prescribed oral cancer drugs, *if* they are covered at all, will require out-of-pocket cost-sharing by patients ranging from 26 to 35 percent of the drugs' prices.[45]

• As for integrity and reliability, the MMA's private offerings have been tarnished by many unscrupulous practices, enabled by minimal government oversight, including deceptive marketing techniques, falsifying signatures on applications, even to the point of criminal behavior (e.g., agents enrolling dead people from information lifted from their Medicare records).[46,47]

• A 2008 GAO study found that private Medicare plans pocketed $1.3 billion in profits in 2006 that should have been paid out in extra benefits to enrollees.[48]

• The Medicare Payment Advisory Commission (MedPAC) has concluded that taxpayers pay more than $3 for every $1 in "extra benefits" provided by Medicare Private Fee-for-Service plans and $2 for such benefits by Medicare PPOs.[49]

### • *Proton Beam Therapy*

As we saw in Chapter 4, there is an "arms race" going on around the country for construction of proton centers in or around hospitals, very large and complex facilities costing some $125 million and involving ongoing operational costs of about $15 million a year. The National Association for Proton Therapy (NAPT), founded in 1990, actively advocates for proton therapy as "the voice of the proton community." Vendors and investment firms are vigorously promoting proton centers as the golden path to new profits. ProCure Treatment Centers is a leading company involved in financing, building and operating proton centers. It offers hospitals and physicians a small ownership stake in facilities as well as a part of profits while directing the treatments. There are obvious conflicts of interest with these kinds of arrangements. Dr. Timothy Williams, former co-chairman of the health policy committee of the American Society for Therapeutic Radiology and Oncology, has recently stated:...

"the profession is threatening to debase itself if doctors are building centers for the money or competitive advantage. "[50]

The NAPT is a dedicated advocate for proton therapy, as indicated by these statements on its Fact Sheet on its Web site:[51]

• "Most precise form of radiation treatment available today. Destroys primary tumor site, leaves surrounding healthy tissue and organs intact and unharmed."

• "Is non-invasive and painless. Maintains a patient's quality-of-life during treatment process as an outpatient. Patients continue with normal activities during treatment. Play golf, tennis, swim, walk, run, workout in a gym, or go on a 'radiation vacation.' "

Despite the hype, however, this is one more example of market forces driving new technology before science has caught up with the market. While there is general consensus that proton therapy is effective, and is an advance over other radiation therapy for cancers of the head, neck and spine, as well as cancers in children, there is no solid evidence as yet that it will be better for other more common cancers. With doctors standing to benefit every time the machines are used, it is likely that it will be oversold and overused for such cancers as prostate cancer without evidence of added clinical benefit over other kinds of treatment. What we do know, however, is that proton therapy will be more expensive, will further raise the costs of cancer care, and that questions of its potential improved clinical outcomes will remain unanswered for years to come.

Do doctors let money cloud their understanding of the benefits and limits of proton therapy? Upton Sinclair said it best: "It is difficult to get a man to understand something when his salary depends upon his not understanding it."

As financial implications of this new technology become more clear, we are already seeing a push-back by state regulators in Michigan and Illinois, where certificates-of-need may be withheld from construction of duplicative proton centers.[52]

### 3. Prices Are Set at "Whatever You Can Get Away With"

Much of the health care industry is investor-owned, whether hospitals, drug and medical device manufacturers, imaging centers, or insurers. As such, they are obligated to their shareholders to maximize profits and returns to investors. As we have also seen, the "not-for-profits" also have wide latitude to independently set prices to what the traffic will bear. And health care is not the same as other commodities, a point that many economists seem to miss. Cancer patients and their families see little alternative but to try to pay whatever costs are involved to get care for cancer, no matter what the prices are.

A bit of history explains some of the reasons for the price-setting latitude of providers and suppliers. As the largest payer in the country, Medicare was enacted in 1965 through a political compromise involving three major industries – medical, hospital, and insurance – which were initially opposed to the program. In order to gain their support, regulatory authority was avoided over the practice of medicine, and Blue Cross, as the lead intermediary, was contracted by Medicare to deal with providers. Permissive and generous reimbursement arrangements were made, with Blue Cross in a privileged position to set rules and procedures favorable to providers.[53] Fiscal intermediaries were authorized to determine whether claims were to be covered, whether they were necessary, and whether charges were *reasonable* and *customary*. Prices soon went up. In 1966, the first year of operation for Medicare, physicians raised their fees by 7.8 percent (more than twice the consumer price index that year) while average daily service charges in hospitals climbed by 21.9 percent.[54]

Over the years, big regional variations in reimbursement have become well entrenched, procedures have received much higher reimbursement than cognitive services (face-to-face evaluative and listening time by physicians with patients). Many services have been approved for coverage by local intermediary offices with lax criteria. As a result, there is wide variation in Medicare spending from one part of the country to another. As an example, per capita Medicare spending in 2000 was $10,550 in Manhattan, New York compared to $4,823 in Portland, Oregon, even after adjusting for age, sex and race. By 2006, Medicare spent about $16,000 a year for each Medicare beneficiary in Miami, double that in San Francisco.[55] One important revelation: the extra money spent in Manhattan netted *no* improvement in quality of care.[56] In high-spending areas, providers regularly game the system by increasing the frequency of specialist visits, the number of hospitalizations, and the use of ICUs. In these ways, reimbursement patterns have distorted the practice of medicine, and contributed to maldistribution of physicians by specialty, enticing them not to where they are needed but to the most lucrative practices. In an interesting twist, the quality of care in higher-reimbursed areas with more specialists has actually *dropped* by permitting more inappropriate and unnecessary care.[57]

Here are just two examples in cancer care that illustrate the extent of this permissive environment:

• In 2006 Genentech set the price of its drug Avastin at about $100,000 a year based on "the value of innovation and the value of new therapies," according to Dr. Susan Desmond-Hellmann, then president of product development.[58] The drug industry always argues that it needs high prices to fund innovation, but the industry's track record shows that it spends about three times as much on marketing and administrative costs as on research and development.[59]

• The "not-for-profit" Carilion Health System in Virginia charges $4,727 for a colonoscopy (4 to 6 times what others charge in the area) and $1,606 for a CT scan of the neck (versus $675 by a local imaging center).[60]

Concerning price-setting in health care, Peter Lindert, Professor of Economics at the University of California Davis with a special interest in public health issues, has this to say: "Prices are whatever you can get away with."[61]

## 4. Perverse Incentives Permeate the System

The cancer care market is rife with perverse incentives that raise costs and maximize profits for facilities, providers, drug manufacturers, and related industries. Conflicts of interest abound throughout, as illustrated by these examples.

### • *Overuse of Imaging Services*

According to Dr. Christopher Ullrich, Chairman of the American College of Radiology (ACR) Managed Care Committee, the costs of imaging procedures have been soaring in double digits, even by as much as 20 to 30 percent year after year. Imaging centers have proliferated as cash cows. The greater Pittsburgh area, population about 3.3 million, has 120 MRI units. Canada, a country 10 times its size by population, has less than twice as many. Many of these centers are owned by physicians who self-refer their own patients for imaging procedures. There is a system for accrediting imaging providers through the ACR and other institutions. Yet less than half of imaging providers have accreditation.[62]

Overuse of imaging services has not led to better outcomes for patients. Dr. Elliot Fisher, from his base at the Center for Evaluative Clinical Sciences at Dartmouth Medical School observes: "We have communities with half as many scanners as those in other parts of the country, and their outcomes are just as good, and in some cases better, than communities spending twice as much on imaging."[63]

In an attempt to rein in overuse of CT, MRI and PET scans, the ACR has become a vocal critic of self-referral. Some insurers are developing their own accreditation program

(UnitedHealthcare), while others (Empire BlueCross BlueShield of New York) are contracting with a national management firm to increase oversight.[64] Medicare has reduced reimbursement of MRI scans by an average of 38 percent, a move strongly opposed by providers and industry (e.g., General Electric, Siemens AG, Toshiba Corp).[65] Medicare is also considering banning its payments for some self-referred services. Self-referred imaging services are estimated to account for $8 billion a year.[66]

### • *Rebates for Chemotherapy and Anemia Drugs*

A profit-making scheme has been going on over the last decade involving two of the world's largest drug companies and oncologists, with entangled conflicts of interest of which most patients are unaware. At issue are chemotherapy and anti-anemia drugs that are injected or given intravenously in oncologists' offices. Rebates are given to treating oncologists by the drug companies based on the volume of drugs purchased and whether they use one company's products exclusively. The head-to-head battle over market share of anti-anemia drugs by Amgen (with its Aranesp and Epogen) and Johnson & Johnson (Procrit) shows how this works.

Sales representatives from the companies actively promote the financial advantages of rebates to oncology practices. Oncologists purchase the drugs in bulk, bill Medicare or private insurers for their costs and services, and receive rebates from the drug manufacturers over and above the reimbursement from the government or private insurers. This scheme involves hundreds of millions of dollars annually. One oncology practice in the Pacific Northwest, with six oncologists, received $1.8 million in rebates in one year. This practice is widespread in the U.S., involving about a million patients a year receiving chemotherapy and kidney dialysis.[67]

The drugs are often given without solid clinical indications, and at higher doses, despite growing concerns over their safety. Several trials in recent years have shown that they increase the risks of heart attacks and strokes, and may also worsen survival from cancer. Despite these risks and perhaps because of these incentives, cancer patients in the U.S. are three times as likely to be given these drugs, and at higher doses, than their counterparts in Europe. In an effort to curb this practice, Medicare has taken the lead in reducing its reimbursements to oncologists. The impact has been huge, and the sales of some drugs (e.g. Amgen's Aranesp) have fallen precipitously.[68,69]

## 5. Markets and Industry Compromise the Integrity of Cancer Research

One might think that markets have little to do with cancer research, but unfortunately that is not the case. Conflicts of interest between researchers and industry play a major role in the kinds of research that are undertaken, the integrity of research design, and whether and how their results are reported. Markets and industry can compromise the quality of cancer research in a number of ways, mostly below the radar screen of public awareness.

These are some of the common ways by which research is negatively influenced.[70]

- undertaking research subjects that are most likely to give positive results for the industry sponsor
- designing the research protocol to favor the sponsor's product (e.g., not comparing against a placebo or a credible comparative group, avoiding head-to-head comparison with a competitor's product, changing primary outcomes in the middle of a study if the results are trending against the sponsor's product, and using the FDA's "low bar" for a successful outcome – that a product only be comparable, not superior to a competitor drug)
- stopping trials early or running them longer than the initial protocol
- non-transparency of data analysis, controlled by the industry sponsor
- publication bias, whereby favorable studies are published, only some outcomes may be reported, and studies with negative results are suppressed
- ghostwriting by industry insiders of articles for publication, often denying co-investigators access to all of the results

About 57 percent of all clinical research is funded by industry, about double that by the National Institutes of Health (28 percent).[71] Conflicts-of-interest (COIs) of investigators with industry sponsors exist at many levels: speaking, honoraria, consulting fees, even insider-trading with Wall Street. A 1999 regulation has required the FDA to identify and mitigate the impacts of financial COIs among researchers who conduct clinical trials of drugs, biologics and medical devices. But a January 2009 report by the Department of Health and Human Services' Office of Inspector General (OIG) found that oversight by the FDA is still very lax in this area. As examples, almost 42 percent of the 118 applications receiving FDA approval in 2007 lacked complete financial information and neither the FDA nor trial sponsors took any corrective action in 20 percent of cases when COIs were identified.[72]

Cancer research fits the overall pattern for other clinical research, and again, conflicts-of-interest are common. As one example, a recent study of participants at the American Society of Clinical Oncology's (ASCO) 2006 meeting found financial conflicts-of-interest among 32 percent of the abstracts submitted and 47 percent of the speakers. These findings are picked up regularly by the media for wide dissemination. As another example, a recent study of papers published in the *Journal of Clinical Oncology* found that at least one financial conflict-of-interest was disclosed in 69 percent of clinical trials and 51 percent of editorials.[73]

Here are four instances that illustrate the extent to which conflicts-of-interest can make us question the integrity of some cancer research.

- A recent study of 56 cancer research articles published in 2003 looked at reports that received industry funding and reports that didn't. Of those disclosing industry funding, fully 84 percent of the reports were favorable to the product studied. When no funding was received, the percentage of favorable reports dropped to 54 percent. Research sponsored by industry was also much more likely to have no comparison arm (66 percent versus 33 percent).[74]
- A remarkable "breakthrough" report published in the prestigious *New England Journal of Medicine (NEJM)* in October, 2006 claimed that annual CT scans of smokers and former smokers could detect small lung cancers when cure was still possible, preventing as many as 80 percent of the 160,000 deaths each year from lung cancer.[75] The problem, however, is that the

researchers did not disclose their sources of funding – including more than \$3.6 million from the deceptively named Foundation for Lung Cancer: Early Detection, Prevention & Treatment (funded by the tobacco industry!). Dr. Claudia Henschke, a professor of radiology at Weill Cornell Medical College in New York, was president of this foundation and the lead author of the article.[76]

Many oncologists gave this report no credibility. Dr. Jerome Kassirer, former editor of the *New England Journal of Medicine* and author of the excellent book *On The Take: How Medicine's Complicity With Big Business Can Endanger Your Health*, observed: [the tobacco industry] "wants to show that lung cancer is not so bad as everybody thinks because screening can save people, and that's outrageous."[77]

Embarrassed by the lack of disclosure by the authors, Dr. Jeffrey Drazen, editor-in-chief of the *NEJM*, added: "In the seven years that I've been here, we have never knowingly published anything supported by a cigarette maker."[78] And of course, just think of the potential future market for diagnostic imaging equipment if research of this kind were to gain acceptance.

• Among 90 drugs approved by the FDA between 1998 and 2000 included in a recent statistical analysis, only 394 of 909 clinical trials were ever published in a peer-reviewed journal; only one in five clinical trials for cancer is ever disclosed in a medical journal.[79]

• Researchers are often approached by Wall Street interests, especially hedge fund representatives or their intermediaries, seeking information about the status or preliminary results of clinical trials underway. Physicians typically receive \$300 to \$500 an hour for advice and information. Some stock analysts may even pose as physicians conducting a trial.[80] One well-known researcher at Cedars-Sinai Comprehensive Cancer Center in Los Angeles is regularly offered (but rejects) \$1,000 to \$1,500 for a half-hour talk with an investor.[81] In one instance, a potential new drug for lung cancer was being found ineffective during trials. Researchers broke their confidentiality agreements and leaked this information to Wall Street investment interests. Biotech stock traders then promptly "sold short" on the sponsor's stock, driving its price way down, and later taking large profits from the stock's decline.[82]

## Rigged Market Justice Versus Social Justice: Can They Co-Exist?

As the foregoing makes clear, powerful corporate interests rule health care in a deregulated marketplace in this country. As with other health care services, cancer care has become a big business cash cow, with potentially large rewards for industry, providers, and investors. The business model pursues profit and financial bottom lines for those who can pay while opposing external regulatory efforts. Under the rules of market justice, health care is allocated by individual resources and choices with little sense of collective obligation or the need for a government role. It is based on principles of individualism, personal effort, self-interest, and voluntary behavior.[83]

Social justice takes an entirely different approach, allocating goods and services by the individual's needs, in this case medical care. It requires equity and ensured access to care through some kind of universal coverage. We have two good examples of social justice within our present health care system – traditional (unprivatized) Medicare and the Veterans Administration.

These two contrasting approaches do not co-exist well. Market justice leads to tiering of health care, where levels of care received depend on one's ability to pay. If they cannot pay, many sick people are excluded from the benefits of necessary care. As a result, they have more advanced disease when recognized, have higher morbidity, and shorter survival. Markets make cancer care for our population worse, and encourage large amounts of inappropriate, unnecessary and even harmful care.

Dr. Peter Budetti, a physician, attorney and chairperson of the Department of Health Administration and Policy at the University of Oklahoma Health Sciences Center, brings us this perspective about health care and justice:

"Health care has become a valuable commodity that created enormously influential vested commercial interests with little motive to abandon market justice. Medicine, which might have played a role in promoting social justice, has not done so, and has been transformed by the imperatives of market justice. Fragmented and struggling to come to terms with externally imposed pressures, medicine is losing both its political force and moral compass. The medicalization of health has simultaneously enhanced the investment in health care goods and services while distracting clinicians and policy makers from attention to the needs for health promotion and disease prevention and constraining the capacity to meet the expanding challenges to public health. Market justice may have outlived its role in U.S. health care."[84]

Joseph Stiglitz, Ph.D., Nobel Laureate in Economics and former chief economist at the World Bank, has this to say about markets:

"Markets do not lead to efficient outcomes, let alone outcomes that comport with social justice. As a result, there is often good reason for government intervention to improve the efficiency of the market. Just as the Great Depression should have made it evident that the market does not work as well as its advocates claim, our recent Roaring Nineties should have made it self-evident that the pursuit of self-interest does not necessarily lead to overall economic efficiency."[85]

If, as Stiglitz points out above, markets are poor dispensers of social justice generally, then it should be clear that the medical marketplace we have reviewed here is especially far distant from any goals of social justice, or for that matter any goals of winning the war on cancer. We need a system that deploys resources to heal as many people as possible. But we are hobbled by a market where consolidation limits competition; profits trump service; prices are set by whatever companies can get away with; nonprofits focus on profit at the expense of caring for those in need; perverse incentives distort decisions about dispensing care; and distortions in research skew our understanding of the value of drugs and therapies. When these factors are viewed collectively, it is easy to see that the medical marketplace, far from providing us with a health care system that better serves the public interest, is actually an obstacle in its own right – and a formidable one at that – to achieving that goal.

The key issue boils down to what should be the role of government in reconciling these opposing systems of justice, and particularly, how should health care and cancer care be financed? That leads us to the next chapter.

# References:

1.  Keehan S, Sisko A, Truffer C, et al. Health spending projections through 2017: the baby-boom generation is coming to Medicare. *Health Affairs Web Exclusive* W145-W155, February 26, 2008.
2.  Comment by McCanne D in Quote-of-the-Day, don@mccanne.org, February 26, 2008.
3.  Gingrich N. *Saving Lives & Saving Money: Transforming Health and Health-care.* Washington, DC. The Alexis de Tocqueville Institution. 2003, pp 81-2.
4.  Callahan D, Wasunna AA. *Medicine and the Market: Equity v. Choice.* Baltimore, The Johns Hopkins Press, 2006, p 270.
5.  Arrow KJ. Uncertainty and the welfare economics of medical care. *American Economic Review* 53: 941-73, 1963.
6.  Ibid # 2, p 38.
7.  Evans RG. Going for the gold: The redistributive agenda behind market-based health care reform. *J Health Polit Policy Law* 22: 427, 1997.
8.  Nichols LM, et al. Are market forces strong enough to deliver efficient health care systems? Confidence is waning. *Health* Affairs 23 (2): 8-21, 2004.
9.  Stein L. Pulling the plug. *Metro* Silicon Valley's weekly newspaper. September 20, 2002.
10. Associated Press. Study: Health insurers are near monopolies. April 18, 2006.
11. Graboyes RF. The impact of health insurance mergers on healthcare costs. Washington, DC: National Federation of Independent Business, August 7, 2008.
12. Robinson JC. Consolidation and the transformation of competition in health insurance. *Health Affairs* 23 (6): 11-24, 2004.
13. Kronick R, Goodman DC, Weinberg J, et al. The marketplace in health care reform. The demographic limitations of managed competition. *N Engl J Med* 328: 148, 1993.
14. AMA. Anthem WellPoint: the doctors' friend. *AMA News* May 19, 2008.
15. Geyman JP. *The Corrosion of Medicine: Can The Profession Reclaim Its Moral Legacy?* Monroe, ME: Common Courage Press, 2008, p37.
16. Chen J, et al. Do "America's Best Hospitals" perform better for acute myocardial infarction? *N Eng J Med* 340: 286, 2003.
17. Hartz AJ, et al. Hospital characteristics and mortality rates. *N Engl J Med* 321: 1720, 1989.
18. Kover C, Gergen PJ. Nurse staffing levels and adverse events following surgery in U.S. hospitals. *Image J Nurs Scholarsh* 30:315, 1998.
19. Silverman EM, et al. The association between for-profit hospital ownership and

increased Medicare spending. *N Engl J Med* 341: 420, 1999.

20. Woolhandler S, Himmelstein DU. Costs of care and administration at for-profit and other hospitals in the United States. *N Engl J Med* 36: 769, 1997.

21. Yuan Z. The association between hospital type and mortality and length of stay: a study of 16.9 million hospitalized Medicare beneficiaries. *Med Care* 38: 231, 2000.

22. Himmelstein DU, et al. Quality of care in investor-owned vs. not-for-profit HMOs. *JAMA* 282: 159, 1999.

23. HMO honor roll. *U.S. News & World Report*, October 23, 1997, p 62.

24. Kuttner R. The American health care system: Wall Street and health care. *N Engl J Med* 340: 664, 1999.

25. Harrington C, et al. Does investor-ownership of nursing homes compromise the quality of care? *Am J Public Health* 91 (9): 1, 2001.

26. Wrich J. *Brief Summary of Audit Findings of Managed Behavioral Health Services*. Chicago: J Wrich & Associates, 1998.

27. Munoz R. How health care insurers avoid treating mental illness. *San Diego Union Tribune*, May 22, 2002.

28. Himmelstein DU, Woolhandler S. Privatization in a publicly funded health care system: the U.S. experience. *Int J Health Serv* 38 (3): 413, 2008.

29. Pollack A. Gene testing questioned by regulators. *New York Times,* June 26, 2008: C1.

30. Helliker K. Nicotine fix. Behind antismoking policy, influence of drug industry. *Wall Street Journal*, February 8, 2007: A 1.

31. O'Connell V. Philip Morris readies global tobacco blitz. *Wall Street Journal,* January 29, 2008: A 1.

32. Weissman R. Corporate Focus. The 10 worst corporations of 2008. *The Progressive Populist* 15 (2), February 1, 2009, p 12.

33. Reuters. Philip Morris International Inc. (PMI) presents at J P Morgan Global Tobacco Conference, June 27, 2008.

34. Elliott S. Advertising. A new Camel brand is dressed to the nines. *New York Times,* February 15, 2007.

35. Wayne A. Tobacco industry faces formidable opponent: support for SCHIP expansion. *CQ Today* – Health. November 14, 2007.

36. Har J. Health plan gets burned after state's costliest race. *The Oregonian* November 7, 2007.

37. Martinez B. Nonprofit hospitals leave the city for greener pastures. *Wall Street Journal*, October 14, 2008: A 1.

38. Martinez B, Carreyrou J. Minority of tax-exempt hospitals provide most charity care. *Wall Street Journal*, February 13, 2009: A3.

39. Hayes RM. Choice of prescription drug and Medicare health plans for 2009. New York: Medicare Rights Center, September 25, 2008.

40. Medicare Rights Center. Clean house. *Asclepios* 8 (10), March 6, 2008.

41. Medicare Rights Center. Turn off the spigot. *Asclepios* 8 (48): December 4, 2008.

42. Medicare Rights Center. *Medicare Watch* 11 (20), September 30, 2008.

43. Kaiser Daily Health Policy Report, January 15, 2009.

44. Ibid # 41.

45. Medicare Rights Center. Drug plans raise cost, restrict access for cancer meds. *Medicare Watch* 11 (26): December 23, 2008.

46. Pear R. Insurer faces reprimand in Medicare marketing case. *New York Times* May 15, 2007: A 14.

47. Williamson E, Lee C. Medicare hard-sell. Abusive tactics found in sales tactics. *Washington Post National Weekly Edition*, May 21-27, 2007: p 24.

48. Medicare Rights Center. First steps. *Asclepios* 8 (49), December 11, 2008.

49. Medicare Rights Center. Scalped! *Asclepios* 8 (50), December 18, 2008.

50. Pollack A. High-tech cancer fight brings big profit. *New York Times* December 26, 2007: A22.

51. Web site for National Association of Proton Therapy (NAPT), accessed October, 19, 2008.

52. Pollack A. States limit costly sites for cancer radiation. *New York Times* May 1, 2008: C4.

53. Oberlander J. *The Political Life of Medicare*. Chicago: University of Chicago Press. 2003, pp 108-11.

54. Marmor TR. *The Politics of Medicare*. New York. Aldine Publishing Company, 1970, p 86.

55. Fisher ES, Bynum JP, Skinner JS. Slowing the growth of health care costs. *N Engl J Med* 360 (9): 849-52, 2009.

56. Dartmouth Atlas of Healthcare Project Web site. (Accessed October 3, 2003) at http://www.dartmouthatlas.org/annals/fisher03.

57. Wennberg JB, Fisher ES, Skinner JS. Geography and the debate over Medicare reform. *Health Affairs Web Exclusive* W96-W114, February 13, 2002.

58. Berenson A. A cancer drug shows promise, at a price that many can't pay. *New York Times* February 15, 2006.

59. Reinhardt UE. Perspectives on the pharmaceutical industry. *Health Affairs* 20 (5): 136, 2001.

60. Carreyrou J. Nonprofit hospitals flex pricing power. *Wall Street Journal* August 28, 2008: A1.

61. Lazarus D. Medical pricing makes the head spin. *Los Angeles Times,* September 7, 2008.

62. Butcher L. Payers seek to rein in radiology costs. *Oncology Times*, June 25, 2007, pp 43-5.

63. Perrone M. MRI, x-ray firms fight Medicare cuts. *Arizona Daily Star,* June 26, 2007.

64. Ibid # 62.

65. Ibid # 63.

66. Armstrong D. Medicare moves to cut 'self-referral' practice. *Wall Street Journal* September 12, 2007: B1.

67. Berenson A. Perverse incentives limit any savings in treating cancer. *New York Times,* June 12, 2007: C1.

68. Ibid # 67.

69. Chase M. Amgen navigates crisis over drug. *Wall Street Journal* March 10, 2008: B1.
70. Ibid # 15, pp 130-5.
71. Moses H, Dorsey ER, Mathesen DHM, et al. Financial anatomy of biomedical research. *JAMA* 294 (11): 1333-42, 2005.
72. Kuehn BM. Report: FDA exerts too little oversight of researchers' conflicts of interest. *JAMA* 301 (7): 709-10, 2009.
73. Goodman A. Study finds increasing financial conflicts of interest in abstracts and among speakers and planners of ASCO annual meetings, as well as in *JCO* articles. *Oncol Times*, June 25, 2007, pp 48-9.
74. Riechelmann RP, Wang L, O'Carroll A, et al. Disclosure of conflicts of interest by authors of clinical trials and editorials in oncology. *J Clin Oncol* 25 (29): 4642-47, 2007.
75. Peppercorn J, Blood E, Winer E, et al. Association between pharmaceutical involvement and outcomes in breast cancer clinical trials FNR HREF. *Cancer* 109 (7): 1239-46, 2007.
76. Henschke CI, Yankelevitz DF, Libby DM, et al. Survival of patients with Stage I lung cancer detected on CT scanning. *N Engl J Med* 355 (17): 1763-71, 2006.
77. Harris G. Cigarette company paid for lung cancer study. *New York Times*, March, 26, 2008: A 1.
78. Ibid # 77.
79. Hotz RL. What you didn't know about a drug can hurt you: Untold numbers of clinical-trial results go unpublished; those that are made public can't always be believed. *Wall Street Journal,* December 12, 2008: A16.
80. Anand G, Smith R. Trial heat: biotech analysts strive to peek inside clinical tests of drugs. *Wall Street Journal*, August 8, 2002: A1.
81. Saul S, Anderson J. Doctors links with investors raise concerns. *New York Times,* August 16, 2005: A1.
82. Heath P, Timmerman L. Drug researchers leak secrets to Wall Street. *The Seattle Times,* August 7, 2005: A1.
83. Dorfman L, Wallack L, Woodruff K. More than a message. *Health Educ Behav* 32 (3): 320-36, 2005.
84. Budetti P. Market justice and US health care. *JAMA* 299 (1): 94, 2008.
85. Stiglitz JE. Evaluating economic change. *Daedalus* 133/3, Summer, 2004.

CHAPTER 9

# Financing Cancer Care: What Are the Options?

"The significant problems we face cannot be solved at the same level of thinking we were at when we created them."
—Albert Einstein (1879-1955)

"Nothing is more difficult than to introduce a new order because the innovator has for enemies all those who have done well under the old conditions and lukewarm defenders in those who may do well under the new."
—Niccolo di Bernardo Machiavelli (1469-1527)

Recall from the Preface the current national campaign by the American Cancer Society (ACS) directed to expanding access to cancer care for all Americans. The ACS has proposed a goal of 4 As for insurance coverage that is *adequate, affordable, available,* and *administratively simple.* As national volunteer president of the ACS in 2007, Dr. Richard Wender had this to say:

"The American Cancer Society believes that, after tobacco use, lack of access to quality health care in the United States could be the biggest barrier to continued progress in the fight against cancer. Cancer is the number one personal health concern of Americans. Reducing suffering and death from cancer may only truly be possible if all Americans are able to visit their doctor for regular check ups, early detection screening tests and prompt, quality cancer treatment if and when they need it."[1]

John Seffrin, Ph.D., as the national chief executive officer of the ACS, adds:

> "As a member of civil society, we have made tremendous progress in the fight against cancer, but that progress will not continue unless all Americans have access to quality health care. To make the next significant leap, we have to make it easier for Americans to get the tests and treatments they need to fight cancer. It's a battle the American Cancer Society is fighting on behalf of every American – regardless of their financial ability or health care history. Is the choice between losing your life and losing everything really a choice?"[2]

Despite all the various proposals to reform health care financing which have been brought forward by politicians and policy makers, there are really only two basic options: (1) build on our present private-public multi-payer financing system with one or another incremental change, or (2) consolidate health care financing through publicly-financed single-payer national health insurance (NHI). These two approaches offer widely different outcomes concerning the system problems we are facing in access, affordability, quality and equity of health care.

This chapter has two goals: (1) to describe how cancer care is financed now through our multi-payer system, together with brief consideration of how effective future incremental changes might be, and (2) to describe how single-payer financing under NHI will improve care in an otherwise private delivery system, and how we can pay for it.

## Multi-Payer Financing: Now and in the Future

As we have already seen, our present multi-payer approach to financing cancer care is a disjointed mix of private and public payers that quickly forces many patients with cancer into serious financial straits. As Wender noted in a 2007 editorial:

> "The work of the American Cancer Society's national call center shows us the real-life urgency of the problems. The cancer specialists are trained to help cancer patients and their caregivers who call with finance and insurance problems. Unfortunately, there are no options to address the needs of 30%

of the callers. Of those who had options, 7 of 10 found that the options were either unaffordable or inadequate for their medical needs. Our inability to help these individuals obtain and maintain affordable coverage is tragic. The stories of those with inadequate insurance should add another dimension to the health care reform debates. We are least able to assist those individuals who have insurance but who cannot access the services they need because the benefits are not covered, they have reached the limit of the benefits under their plan, or they can no longer pay their share of the cost of services. Clearly, the issues of adequacy, availability, and affordability of coverage are serious problems that must be addressed collectively as we work to fix what is wrong with our health care system."[3]

How do the present payers of cancer care sort out, and what can we expect if we continue with multi-payer financing? Let's take each of the current sources of payment for cancer care in turn.

## Medicare

About three of five cancer patients are 65 years of age or older, so much of their care is covered by Medicare from the outset. In addition, many cancer patients younger than 65, as they confront the high costs of care, end up on Medicare after a two-year wait on Social Security disability. Oncology accounts for about 10 percent of all Medicare expenditures.[4] Part A covers 80 percent of the costs of inpatient cancer care, while Part B covers 80 percent of the costs of approved screening and treatment services. Part D provides partial drug coverage, as previously described, through private Medicare plans.[5]

Faced with continued double-digit increases in the costs of cancer care, Medicare officials are attempting in various ways to put some reasonable brakes on spending while improving quality and reducing waste. These include efforts to reduce or eliminate incentives that encourage more costly treatments when lower-cost approaches can be equivalent or preferable, revising its coverage and reimbursement policies, and promoting wider use of evidence-based clinical practice guidelines.[6] Since the prevalence of cancer increases sharply with age,[7] future projections of the costs of cancer care are further challenged by the aging of our population. By 2030, the number of Americans over age 65 will double and the number over 85 will quadruple. We can expect that these pressures will require a much greater role by Medicare (or whatever financing mechanism is in place at that time) in negotiating prices of services, using economic analysis to evaluate alternative approaches to screening and treatment, and eliminating billions in overpayments to private Medicare plans that only add to their profits without significant return in benefits.

## Private Insurance

As we have already seen in earlier chapters, having health "insurance" all too often amounts to very little protection against the high costs of cancer care. Many insured cancer patients end up being bankrupted by those costs. Insurers have many ways to avoid such high expenditures and "medical losses", including denial of initial coverage on the basis of pre-existing conditions or family history, marketing policies with limited benefits (such as Allstate's "cancer policy" with its $2,000 cap),[8] high deductibles, denial of benefits if "covered", cancellation of coverage, hiking premiums by annual re-underwriting to unaffordable levels, or setting low annual or lifetime caps on benefits. Almost one in three survivors of childhood cancer report difficulty in getting insurance, a rate of difficulty ten times as high as the 3 percent of their siblings.[9] As the costs of chemotherapy drugs go through the roof, insurers have taken to requiring that enrollees pay 20 to 33 percent of the costs of the drugs, often amounting to thousands of dollars a month for Tier 4 drugs such as Avastin. So private insurance frequently provides little security against the costs of cancer care.

Health insurers are large corporate entities that exact a heavy toll on those they insure, as we have seen. It may seem that their size and power mean that they are financially healthy, sustainable, and too big to fail. In fact, however, the industry is on a death march as a result of these eight factors, as documented in my recent book *Do Not Resuscitate: Why the Health Insurance Industry Is Dying, and How We Must Replace It*:[10]

1. Uncontrolled inflation of health care costs, with 31 percent of costs taken up by the inefficiency and waste of the health insurance industry
2. Growing unaffordability of premiums (recall Figure 3.3) and health care; the average premium for employer-based insurance

is now more than $12,000 a year for a family of four, with less coverage each year; since most health policy experts consider that health care expenditures more than 10 percent of family income constitute a financial hardship, families of four now need an annual income of $120,000 just to pay their premiums without hardship, let alone their actual costs of care if they get sick! How can that be sustained?

3. Decreasing levels of coverage in terms of breadth, reliability and value, all of which reduce the desire to purchase the insurance, thereby threatening the business model further

4. Fragmentation and inefficiency among 1,300 private insurers, all using the business model to enroll healthier people and avoid undue "medical losses"

5. Shrinking private insurance markets; only 59 percent of employers sponsor coverage, small businesses avoid coverage if possible, and group coverage is often unaffordable

6. Shift toward privatized public markets in Medicare and Medicaid vulnerable to budget cutbacks

7. Ineffective state and federal regulation, despite a majority of states enacting guaranteed issue and guaranteed renewability laws and all 50 states requiring that some specific benefits be covered, such as screening mammograms

8. Growing economic insecurity and hardship, including for the insured

## TABLE 9.1

## Why Private Health Insurance is Obsolete

- Inefficiencies vs. public-financing
- Fragments risk pools by medical underwriting
- Increasing epidemic of underinsurance
- Excessive administrative and overhead costs
- Profiteering – shareholders trump patients
- Pricing itself out of the market
- Unsustainable and resists regulation

Source: Geyman JP. *Do Not Resuscitate: Why the Health Insurance Industry Is Dying, and How We Must Replace It.* Monroe, ME. Common Courage Press, 2008.

A current example shows how far beyond the reach of family budgets health insurance has gone. In an effort to avoid underinsurance, prevent cherry picking by health insurers and assure adequate benefits, New York State requires insurers to guarantee issue to anyone, regardless of health status. Though they may still be subject to a waiting period of up to one year for certain pre-existing conditions, uninsured New Yorkers can purchase an HMO or HMO/POS plan at any time during the year on the independent market. *But* – annual premiums for family coverage now run from $45,312 to $81,888 for HMO/POS plans (Empire BlueCross BlueShield HMO comes in at $48,792). These rates are not typos! If you are willing to give up full choice of providers and hospitals and stay within an HMO plan, your premiums for family coverage range from only $27,192 to $68,232 a year![12,13] That such premiums are totally unaffordable for most people is shown by Figure 9.1, based on an April 2009 report of a joint national survey by NPR, the Kaiser Family Foundation, and Harvard School of Public Health.[14]

The relentless escalation of the costs of employer-sponsored insurance is taking an ever larger bite out of both employers' and employees' budgets. Annual premiums for family coverage doubled from $5,791 in 1999 to $12,680 in 2009. Employees paid an average of $3,354 for that coverage in 2008 for premiums alone.[15] How can one possibly say that these rates can be sustained?

The dire condition of the health insurance industry is being recognized by some insiders within the industry. As an example, this observation by John Sinibaldi, a highly experienced St. Petersburg, Florida-based health insurance agent, was recently posted to his colleagues on a national health care brokers' forum:

"A huge segment of the American population is simply far too strapped to ever afford the premiums and costs associated with health insurance/health care as it is structured today." [He calls particular attention to the plight of small business and individuals seeking health insurance]: "While the employee of a regional electric utility is complaining about monthly payroll deductions for his family that now exceed $500 or more on a $60,000 annual salary, the longtime employee of a local small electrician is looking at monthly payroll deductions for his family of $1,500 on a $35,000 annual salary. His apprentice is

FIGURE 9.1

# How Much Would Uninsured Be Willing to Pay for Coverage?

AMONG THE 15% OF UNINSURED ADULTS AGES 18-64:
If you were shopping for a health insurance policy, what is the highest amount you would be willing to pay for a monthly premium, that is the amount you pay each month for health insurance?

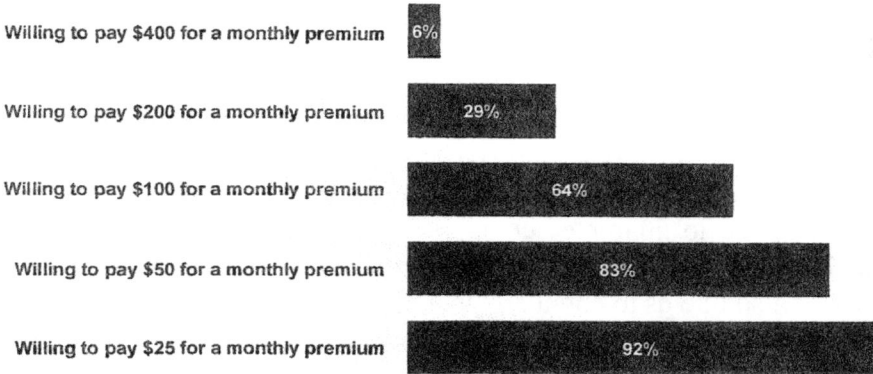

Willing to pay $400 for a monthly premium — 6%

Willing to pay $200 for a monthly premium — 29%

Willing to pay $100 for a monthly premium — 64%

Willing to pay $50 for a monthly premium — 83%

Willing to pay $25 for a monthly premium — 92%

Source: The Public and the Health Care Delivery System. Summary & Chartpack. NPR/ Kaiser Family Foundation/Harvard School of Public Health, April 2009.

Reprinted with permission from the Henry J. Kaiser Family Foundation. The Kaiser Family Foundation is a non-profit private operating foundation, based in Menlo Park, California, dedicated to producing and communicating the best possible information, research and analysis on health issues.

younger, and so is 'fortunate' to have monthly deductions for his family of only $900 on a $20,000 annual salary. The electrician's helper making $9/hr can't afford even half of the premium for just himself. Individuals on personal health insurance policies are also feeling the 'pinch'. Most of my individual clients see increases of 18-25% a year."[16]

Can the private health insurance industry survive? A misguided but firm belief that the market can provide the best care has propelled an endless number of "reforms" intended to "fix" the system. As also described in *Do Not Resuscitate*, over the years these many approaches have included employer and individual mandates, tax credits, state high-risk pools, association health plans, chronic disease management, pay for performance, and information technology.[17] But all of these incremental "reforms" won't rescue a dying industry. At most, they can only prolong the death throes of the industry if enough taxpayer dollars are shoveled toward the insurance companies. Our goal shouldn't be to save a failed private insurance industry but instead to improve and save the lives of patients who need medical care.

The industry's trade group, America's Health Insurance Plans (AHIP), continues to promote its self-serving "reform plan", proposed in 2006, which calls for the federal government to spend about $300 billion over 10 years to expand coverage to all children within 3 years and 95 percent of adults within 10 years.[18] But most of the heavy lifting to cover the sick would be borne by taxpayers through public financing, not by private insurers. The AHIP proposal protects the industry from assuming too much risk by inserting this caveat – any one insurer cannot be expected to guarantee coverage to more than half of one percent of its total enrollment in the individual market.[19] AHIP and its allies would also like us to count any increase in the number of "insured", no matter how skimpy the coverage, as a milestone success without regard to the harms and pain of underinsurance. "Universal health care", then, becomes a propaganda term used by the insurance industry exalting widespread coverage while ignoring that the coverage is inadequate and that the government will still be required to cover most higher-risk people through one or another public program.

We can choose to keep private health insurance alive – if we are willing to spend billions every year to prop it up. But what do we get for this? Throughout the last several chapters, we have seen the woefully inadequate answer. Dr. Marcia Angell, former editor of *The New England Journal of Medicine*, provides a useful thumbnail review of our present predicament:

> "The U.S. system is unique in treating health care as a commodity to be bought and sold in a marketplace. Care is distributed according to the ability to pay, not according to medical need. Private insurers compete by avoiding high-risk individuals, limiting services for those they cover, and, whenever possible, shifting costs to other payers or to patients in the form of high deductibles and co-payments. We have the only health system in the world based on avoiding sick people. It's a chaotic and

fragmented system that requires mountains of paper-work, which is one reason premiums are so high. Employers who offer health benefits react by capping their contributions, so that workers pay more out of pocket and bear the full brunt of premium increases."[20]

## Medicaid

Medicaid can provide some coverage for some cancer patients, but there are many obstacles in their way to qualify for the program. As a federally-aided, state-operated and administered program, it is the largest budget item in most states' budgets, and is on the chopping block more than ever during this economic downturn. Total federal and state Medicaid funding for 2008 was about $339 billion, and its costs are projected to go up by 7.9 percent annually to $647 billion by 2017.[21] About 48 million Americans are on Medicaid, but states are now in a serious budget crunch that is forcing many to make draconian cuts in coverage. Thirty-nine states have frozen or cut Medicaid benefits and/ or payments to physicians. [22]

Even before this economic downturn, many states were cutting Medicaid to the bone. Eligibility and coverage policies vary widely from one state to another, and the federal government has been granting waivers to allow states greater discretion over their programs. In Utah, Medicaid coverage of hospital and specialty care has been eliminated for some Medicaid patients.[23] In Missouri, a family of three must have an annual income less than $3,504 in order to qualify.[24] In February 2008, CMS proposed new rules which give states even more control over their Medicaid benefit packages and increased latitude to impose more cost-sharing on enrollees.[25] In other words, states are being given greater and greater latitude to provide less and less coverage.

Although cancer patients in most states can apply for Medicaid coverage as medically needy even if their incomes are above the states' eligibility limits, they still have to "spend down" by offsetting their "excess income" with medical expenses.[26] We have seen examples in earlier chapters of how extreme this spend-down has to be to qualify for Medicaid. Even after gaining coverage, however, Medicaid patients often find that oncologists refuse to provide chemotherapy in their offices due to low Medicaid reimbursement, referring them on to hospitals.[27] And as we have already seen, by the time cancer patients do get on

Medicaid, they have more advanced cancer and worse outcomes.[28]

## Self-Pay, Out-of-Pocket

Even for those who have health insurance, out-of-pocket expenditures (OOPE) account for a greater portion of cancer care financing all the time. For those fortunate enough to have good initial insurance coverage, they can expect to pay for more OOPE through higher premiums, co-payments, and deductibles, and other costs over the course of their illness. At the other end of the coverage spectrum, the uninsured and other self-pay patients are especially vulnerable to high OOPE for cancer care. They are typically charged much more than their insured counterparts. A 2007 report found that hospitals often bill uninsured and self-pay patients almost 2.5 times the rates charged to insurers. That amounts to more than 3 times what the hospital is allowed to charge Medicare.[29]

As previously noted, many patients with cancer are driven into bankruptcy because of the increasingly high and unaffordable costs of cancer care. The Medical Expenditure Panel Surveys for 1996 and 2003, sponsored by the Agency for Healthcare Research and Quality (AHRQ) examined the financial burden on cancer patients. Almost one-third had expenses more than 10 percent of family income.[30] An earlier study of medical bankruptcy found that one in three who were insured at the onset of their illness lost their insurance over the course of treatment, and that the mean OOPE for cancer patients filing for bankruptcy exceeded $35,000.[31] All present trends in multi-payer financing indicate that OOPE will continue to rise sharply in the future, with no effective mechanism in place for containing the costs of health insurance or health care. This situation has led researchers at the American Cancer Society to ask:

"To what extent do individuals forego treatment or select less than optimal treatment because they are unable to find a health care provider who is willing to provide it or because they are afraid of the level of medical debt that they would incur? As the cost of some new cancer therapies can exceed $100,000 a year, to what extent will availability and type of insurance coverage, as well as individual financial resources, determine who has access to the most effective therapies?"[32]

## Clinical Trials

Cancer patients participating in clinical trials typically have the costs of treatment and laboratory studies covered by the trial's sponsor. But other "routine" costs, such as hospitalizations and outpatient care, are another story. Most insurers refuse coverage for that care on the basis of its being "experimental". Medicare has covered such care since 2001, but coverage by private insurers of "routine" cancer care varies widely from one state to another as a state-by-state battle. This patient's experience illustrates the issue:

*Steffanie, 18, was under treatment for a malignant brain tumor in 2006. After enrolling in a clinical trial, she received a stem cell transplant, which was covered by the trial. But her insurer denied coverage for her subsequent "routine" care as "experimental", which ended up costing her parents almost $500,000. Advocates pushed for passage of a state bill requiring insurers to cover all routine costs of care for cancer patients enrolled in clinical trials. It later passed in the State Senate, but was killed in the House. Steffanie recently died, leaving her family with enormous medical bills.* [33,34]

While clinical trial funding can help some cancer patients with their overwhelming costs of care, it remains a small part of overall cancer financing. Only 3 to 5 percent of all eligible cancer patients are enrolled in clinical trials.[35] And although 63 percent of cancer patients in the U.S. are 65 years of age or older, they account for only 25 percent of patients participating in clinical trials.[36] On the other hand, as we will discuss in a later chapter, much larger enrollment of cancer patients in clinical trials is an important future goal, so that this mechanism can and should assume a greater role in financing cancer care.

## Payment Assistance Programs

There are other resources that can help some cancer patients to pay for some of the costs of their care. As listed in Appendix 2, many state governments, cancer-related organizations and drug companies offer various kinds of patient assistance programs, which may help with co-payments or the cost of drugs. In addition, selected psychosocial services, such as counseling and decision support, are available to patients and their families at no cost, again as listed in the Appendix.

# A Recap of Multi-Payer Financing for Cancer Care

Within our current multi-payer financing system, what kind of coverage can an individual expect if and when he or she gets cancer? From the above and earlier chapters, we can answer that question with just two words – *it depends*. These are some of the things that coverage depends on:

- One's age, pre-existing conditions, family history (perhaps even genetic history), health status, income and employment
- If covered through your employer, coverage further depends on the employer maintaining coverage, keeping your job, level of benefits, fine print in one's policy, income (to afford increasing premiums, co-payments and deductibles), whether or not the insurer denies claims, annual and lifetime caps on benefits, and whether you can understand your options well enough to make informed decisions during annual open-enrollment periods.
- If one loses insurance, such as by changing jobs, illness, accident, or no longer being able to afford coverage, potential public sources of coverage depend on one's age (a child for State Children's Health Insurance Program eligibility?), (65 or older for Medicare?), being a veteran (VA eligibility?), one's home state (Medicaid eligibility if income below the threshold), being able to afford cost-sharing, extent of benefits, and state of the economy (federal and state).

In effect, then, multi-payer financing of cancer care is complex, disjointed, unreliable, insecure, costly, and increasingly unaffordable. The private insurance industry goes to great lengths to avoid covering too many sick people, and is falling on its own sword as a result of its inefficiencies, bureaucratic waste, and profiteering. It has lost the public trust, and should no longer be propped up by government subsidies.

This observation by Dr. Sidney Wolfe, director of Public Citizen's Health Research Group, encapsulates the inherent problems of our present private financing system for health care:

"As unemployment rises, we can expect a decrease in the rate of employer-sponsored insurance. We cannot continue to rely on a 'safety net' that catches only some of the population for some conditions some of the time. We therefore continue to advocate for a single-payer system that would pool all our current health care payments and use them to leverage a fairer and more efficient system that is comprehensive in coverage, that husbands resources, and better allocates health care expenditures. Until we have health care that covers all and is equitable in access and cost, we will not have a society that honors life, secures liberty, and promotes the pursuit of happiness."[37]

## Single-Payer Financing Through National Health Insurance

Our persistent challenge is how to ensure universal access to care, improve its efficiency, quality and fairness, and still make it affordable and sustainable. We have seen the immense and growing problems of the private insurance industry. We will soon be forced to adopt an alternative to a failing system, whether the industry likes it or not, and we can learn from other countries' experiences in doing so.

Most industrialized countries around the world have one or another form of social insurance assuring access to health care for their entire populations. These countries include most of Europe, the United Kingdom, Canada, New Zealand, Taiwan, and others. They all spend much less than we do on health care, and most have better outcomes of care than in the U.S. Although the details vary considerably from one country to another, most have private delivery systems. Support for public financing in these countries is generally very high, and none would trade their systems for ours. In return for their tax support of their universal coverage system, taxpayers gain relief from high out-of-pocket costs when they get sick, as well as the peace of mind that serious illness won't bring financial ruin, something that private insurance cannot offer. Robert Evans, Ph.D., health economist at the University of British Columbia's Centre for Health and Policy Research, sums up the differences between public and private financing this way:

"Public health insurance performs two critical functions that private insurers cannot. They redistribute resources and contain costs. Whether one celebrates or deplores the result, this is what they do. Universal, compulsory, tax-financed health care systems base access to care on need, not ability to pay, while imposing the cost burden in proportion to tax liability. This benefits the unhealthy and unwealthy at the expense of the healthy and wealthy. Such systems also have access to more effective cost control mechanisms than are available in private markets. The exceptional American reliance on private insurance lies at the root of both exceptional cost escalation and exceptional inequity."[38]

Enactment of single-payer national health insurance (NHI) through legislation along the lines of H.R. 676 (the Conyers Bill) will transform cancer care overnight into a program that all Americans can depend on. No longer can one's age, pre-existing conditions, family history, health status, income, employment, or home state be reasons to exclude one from coverage. All Americans living in the United States and U.S. Territories will have a United States National Health Insurance (USNHI) card that ensures access to all necessary care – from prevention and screening to diagnosis, treatment, survival care and palliative care – through a reliable program that shares risk across our entire population. Many benefits not covered by today's Medicare will be covered by NHI, including full prescription drug coverage, more extensive outpatient services (including dentistry, chiropractic, mental health services, and substance abuse treatment), nursing home care, and home care.

This family's experience with a private Medicare plan, as reported to the Medicare Rights Center's Private Health Plan Monitoring Project, illustrates classic differences between the reliability of private and public financing of cancer care.

*"My husband signed up with a private insurance company as a secondary plan and Medicare as primary plan. In fact, we find that the private insurance company is primary. My husband has recently been diagnosed with colon cancer that has spread to his lymph nodes and into his liver. He has had surgery to remove half of his colon and lymph nodes. The doctor has referred him to a cancer center which we find is not in the network, in our area or elsewhere. We have called to have it switched back to traditional Medicare which the center will accept but are told*

*we cannot switch till November which is 6 months from now. We have explained to them that this cannot wait that long – that is half of the time he has been given and they have as much as told us they don't care if he dies. We feel we have been lied to and now my husband can have no treatment till November. This really isn't fair to him."*[39]

Cost-sharing, whereby the patient pays out of pocket some of the costs of his or her care, will be eliminated under NHI. Health care services will be provided based on medical need, not ability to pay. Patients will be encouraged to seek care earlier, rather than being forced to forego care and end up in Emergency Rooms with more advanced disease. Critics immediately cry out that such a program will break the bank because of overuse of the system and moral hazard. But that has not been a limiting problem in other countries, which instead have gained the advantages of wider access to care with better outcomes. We will discuss that issue more thoroughly in the next chapter.

Cost containment mechanisms will be put in place under NHI. These will include evidence-based coverage policies through a national system based on the latest science deciding what services are sufficiently beneficial and cost-effective to be covered. That will be a far cry from the way coverage decisions are made today. As we have seen, market forces strongly influence what tests, drugs and procedures are brought to market, often with little concern for their benefits or cost-effectiveness. Other cost containment mechanisms will include global budgeting for hospitals, HMOs and other facilities; negotiated prices and fees for providers; and more effective monitoring of utilization and clinical outcomes.

This kind of universal coverage will eliminate much of the inefficiency and waste of the private insurance industry, and actually cost employers and individuals *less* than we are already paying for insurance and health care. Medical loss ratios and shareholder dividends will no longer be the benchmarks of success, but rather population-based measures of access and quality of care. Table 9.2 summarizes the main features of single-payer NHI.

How is all that possible? And is it utopian pie in the sky? These are some of the reasons that make publicly financed NHI, coupled with a private delivery system, solidly realistic and achievable:

TABLE 9.2

# **Main Features of Single-Payer NHI**

| | |
|---|---|
| **Access** | Universal access to all necessary medical care without cost-sharing or other barriers to care; all Americans receive NHI card throughout the country and U.S. Territories |
| **Choice** | Full choice of physicians and other licensed providers, hospital or other facilities in a private delivery system |
| **Benefits** | All medically necessary care, including primary care, emergency care, hospital services, mental health services, prescriptions, eye care, dental care, rehabilitation services, nursing home and home care |
| **Medical Decision-Making** | Clinical decisions made by patients and their physicians, not by invisible clerks and others in today's private insurance bureaucracy |
| **Cost Savings** | About $380 billion a year, mainly due to administrative simplification, monopsony purchasing, and improved access with greater use of preventive services and earlier diagnosis of illness |
| **How Financed** | All federal health program funds, such as Medicare and Medicaid, channeled into NHI program; remaining needs from payroll tax on employers (about 7 percent) and income tax on individuals (about 2 percent, but progressive by income) |
| **Private insurance** | Eliminate private insurance duplicating NHI coverage; retraining programs for those losing jobs in such areas as marketing, eligibility determination, and billing |
| **Administration** | NHI program administered by public or quasi-public agency as a single insurance plan with federal, state and regional boards; all costs paid by these agencies without billings to patients; global operating budgets for hospitals, nursing homes, HMOs and other providers; separate allocation of capital funds; adjustable budgets based on demographics, legitimate delivery costs, inflation, and beneficial new technologies |
| **Accountability** | Transparent public accountability; elected representation on federal, state and regional boards for governance and priority-setting |

Source: Adapted and updated from Himmelstein, DU, Woolhandler, S. National Health Insurance or incremental reform: Aim high, or at our feet? *Am J Public Health* 93 (1): 31, 2003.

1. **NHI will assure universal coverage, which no previous incremental efforts have provided.**

   The present multi-payer financing system takes up 31 percent of the health care dollar,[40] with 1,300 private insurers competing to enroll the healthiest 80 percent of the population that accounts for only 20 percent of health care costs.[41] As we have seen, those same insurers do their best to flee from covering people who most need insurance. This system will never succeed in covering everybody. For its increasing costs and decreasing coverage, this system is no longer sustainable.

2. **NHI will bring administrative simplification, with much less bureaucracy than we now have.**

   We have seen an exponential growth in bureaucracy among private insurers, as illustrated by expansion of its work force by one-third between 2000 and 2005, even during a period when private insurance enrollment *dropped* by one percent.[42] Most of this growth in work force was involved in the burgeoning industry of "denial management", the industry's term for dealing with irate patients and physicians when claims are denied. With NHI, coverage is uniform for everybody, and administrative processes are greatly simplified.

3. **Because of that simplification, NHI will be more efficient and have lower overhead costs.**

   Administrative overheads are wildly disparate between private and public financing systems. Despite the claims of market advocates, public programs are much more efficient than private programs. For example, Medicare's overhead is only about 3 percent versus commercial carriers' average of about 20 percent and investor-owned Blues' overhead of 26.5 percent;[43] a 2005 report found that the costs of sales, marketing, billing, and other administrative tasks took up about 22 percent of premium revenue of California insurers.[44]

4. **The savings from the simplification are so great that single-payer NHI will not cost more, and will even save money.**

   Continuing savings will come from simplification throughout the system. Just one billing form for physicians, other providers and facilities; the 17,000 different health plans in Chicago will be a thing of the past,[45] as will the 755 different plans for depressed patients in Seattle;[46] no need for marketing costs, since everyone is already covered; and so on. A landmark 2003 study of the administrative costs of our market-driven system showed that paperwork for U.S. health care cost $294.3 billion in 1999; extrapolations over the last 10 years estimate that NHI will save an estimated $380 billion a year from our present administrative costs (that's more than $1,000 a year for every person in this country!).[47] Other major savings will be achieved by bulk purchasing of drugs, medical devices and other supplies through a single purchaser. These savings are not speculative: the VA already accomplishes this, getting a discount on drug prices of more than 40 percent.[48]

5. **As a result of improved access, health disparities will be reduced and the quality of care should increase for the entire population.**

How can that be? Even with no increase in health care funding, quality improvement can be anticipated because people will no longer have financial barriers to care, can seek care earlier, and preventive services will be covered. Our current system has huge incentives for doctors and all providers to follow the money, that is, to locate in areas where their practices will be lucrative. Under a single-payer system, physicians and other providers are paid for every patient they care for because every single one of them is 100% insured. They get paid the same whether they are treating a rich person or someone who is destitute, whether they practice in a wealthy neighborhood or in a low income area. As will be discussed further in the last chapter, gaps in reimbursement between primary care, which is under-reimbursed, and many procedure-oriented specialties, which are over-reimbursed, will be narrowed. In earlier chapters we noted the critical shortage of primary care physicians, as well as their extraordinary value in the front line in the battle against cancer. Only a coordinated system like single-payer can address these shortages.

As we have already seen, it is estimated that up to one-third of health care is either inappropriate, unnecessary, or even harmful.[49] Regional variation studies have also documented that areas of the country that have more specialists and more intense levels of care cost much more, and have worse outcomes of care compared to areas with more primary care physicians and less use of specialist and intensive care services.[50] With NHI, we will have a structure within which to better control what is paid for, eliminating coverage of services that are either inappropriate or unnecessary. Reimbursement reform should also encourage more medical graduates to enter primary care and other shortage specialties.

6. **Single-payer systems contain health care costs better than multi-payer systems.**

   This has been demonstrated by Medicare in this country for over 30 years,[51] by Canada (Figure 9.2),[52] and more recently, by Taiwan.[53] Growth rates of medical expenditures have been found to be slowest in countries with universal health care systems.[54] Once again, the U.S. stands out as "exceptional", but not in the right way!

7. **We can afford NHI; in fact, we can't afford to go on with multi-payer financing!**

   We already have enough money in our health care system to pay for universal coverage through NHI, which will save money and

FIGURE 9.2

## Health Costs as Percent of GDP: United States And Canada 1960-2008

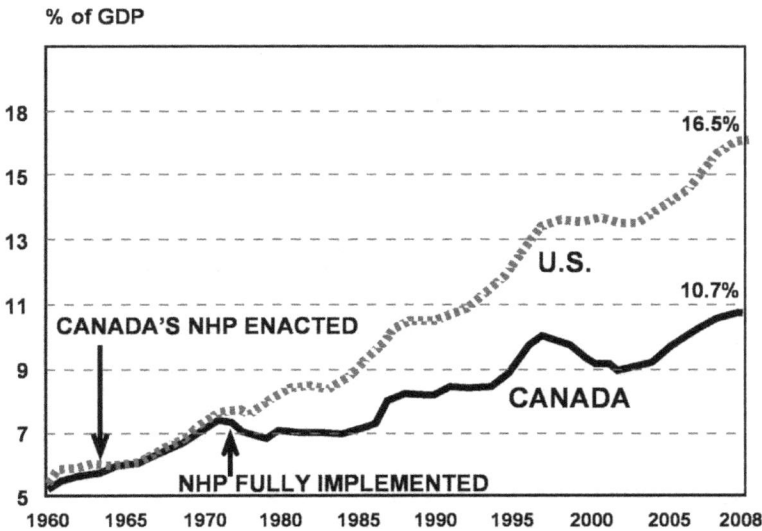

Sources: Woolhandler S, Himmelstein DU. The National Health Program Slideshow Guide, Cambridge, MA. Center for National Health Program Studies; Health care spending to reach $5,170 per person, The Canadian Press, November, 13, 2008. Reprinted with permission

reallocate spending our $2.5 trillion based on medical need, not ability to pay.

Public financing (through taxes, federal health programs, tax exemptions, and disproportionate share payments to hospitals for uncompensated care) now accounts for more than 60 percent of health care funding.[55,56] That is more than total health care spending in countries with universal coverage (Figure 9.3).[57] Employers pay for less than 20 percent of our health care budget with out-of-pocket spending covering the remaining amount.[58]

Under NHI, both employers and taxpayers will pay less than they do now for health insurance. H. R. 676 calls for a payroll tax on employers of about 7.7 percent (less than the average of 8.5 percent that they now pay) and an income tax averaging 2 percent for most taxpayers (higher for those with very high incomes); the 2 percent tax will be more than offset by no longer having to pay larger costs now being paid through insurance premiums, co-payments, deductibles, and other out-of-pocket payments. To put all this in sharper perspective, Table 9.3 shows what taxpayers in three income groups are now paying toward health care, based on estimates by the CBO.[59]

## TABLE 9.3

## What Americans Pay Into the U.S. Health Care System Today

|  |  | Household Income Level | | |
| --- | --- | --- | --- | --- |
|  |  | $25,000 | $50,000 | $75,000 |
| Share and Amount of Income Going to Health Care via Taxes Alone | | 9.0% ($2,425) | 9.8% ($5,300) | 10.7% ($8,633) |
| Share and Amount of Total Wage Packet Going to Health Care for Households With Insurance | Individual | 22.0% ($6,904) | 16.8% ($9,779) | 15.4% ($13,112) |
| | Family | 37.2% ($14,531) | 26.4% ($17,406) | 22.3% ($20,749) |

Source: Harrison JA. Paying more, getting less. *Dollars & Sense*. May/June 2008.

FIGURE 9.3

# U.S. Public Spending Per Capita for Health is Greater Than Total Spending in Other Nations

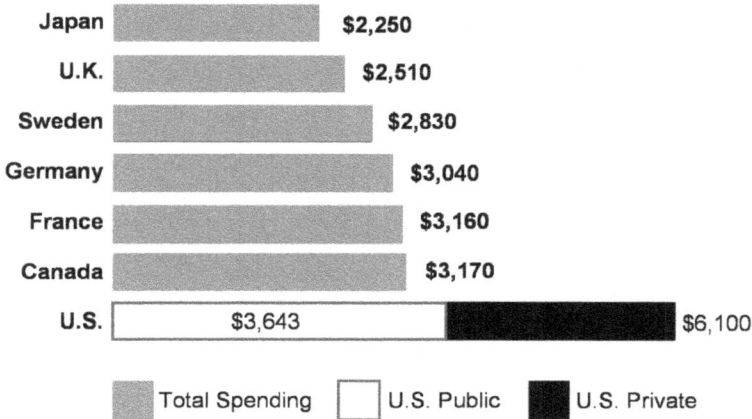

| Japan | $2,250 |
| U.K. | $2,510 |
| Sweden | $2,830 |
| Germany | $3,040 |
| France | $3,160 |
| Canada | $3,170 |
| U.S. | $3,643 ... $6,100 |

Total Spending · U.S. Public · U.S. Private

Note: Public includes benefit costs for government employees and tax subsidy for private insurance. Data are for 2004. Source: Author Compilation

Source: Woolhandler S. Interview. Unhealthy solutions: Private insurance, high cost and the denial of care. *Multinational Monitor* September/October, 2008, p 38. Reprinted with permission.

8. **NHI is a better fit with traditional American values than our present market-based system.**

This claim will elicit a firestorm of protest from market advocates and entrepreneurs, but let's look at that notion a bit.

As argued in my earlier book *Do Not Resuscitate*, national health insurance is not a liberal or conservative issue, but an American issue. It's about having an efficient and fair system, one that provides more choice and value of care for all Americans, eliminates waste, helps American business to become competitive again in a global economy, is fiscally responsible for individuals and society, and is sustainable. Based on all of the evidence brought together in this book, single-payer NHI is our best match with our basic values. Our present multi-payer financing system fails the test on all counts, as shown in Table 9.4.[60]

TABLE 9.4

# Alternative Financing Systems and American Values

| TRADITIONAL VALUE | Single-Payer | Multi-Payer |
|---|:---:|:---:|
| Efficiency | ↑ | ↓ |
| Choice | ↑ | ↓ |
| Affordability | ↑ | ↓ |
| Actuarial value | ↑ | ↓ |
| Fiscal responsibility | ↑ | ↓ |
| Equitable | ↑ | ↓ |
| Accountable | ↑ | ↓ |
| Integrity | ↑ | ↓ |
| Sustainable | ↑ | ↓ |

Source: Geyman JP. *Do Not Resuscitate: Why the Health Insurance Industry Is Dying, and How We Must Replace It*. Monroe, ME. Common Courage Press,

## Winners and Losers with NHI

Despite the rhetoric of the last-ditch stakeholders of the status quo, NHI is a win-win for almost everybody. Most importantly, patients and their families can gain access to all necessary care that is more affordable and of better quality than they now have. They gain the security of knowing that care will be available in a stable system. People of all ages will have full access, with free choice of options, within a private delivery system. This will be a true private-public partnership – private health care, public financing.

Business and labor will also win big. Employers will spend less on health care, get a healthier work force, and will be able to better compete in a global economy. As Lee Iacocca, the retired chairman of Chrysler said in 2005: "The U.S. automobile industry spends more per car on health care than on steel." G. Richard Wagoner, Jr., as chairman and CEO of General Motors, added: "Health care costs add $1,500 to the price of GM vehicles. Fix what's broken."[61] Because of the lower health care costs in the Canadian single-payer system, so many jobs in the automobile industry have moved across the border since 2004 that Ontario, not Michigan, has become the largest car-producing region in North America.[62] NHI will directly address this competitive disadvantage by leveling the playing field with competitors in other nations with universal coverage health care systems.

Small business, increasingly unable to provide any insurance at all, will do much better. This example describes typical problems of small business and the positive impact of NHI in helping smaller employers to have an insured and healthier workforce.

*Alliance Packaging is a manufacturing company in the Pacific Northwest with 550 employees. Alliance funds the full cost of its employees' personal health insurance, as well as 50 to 90 percent of their family coverage, depending on their pay level. The insurance coverage is generous, even including dental benefits, with relatively low deductibles and co-payments. But Alliance is struggling to keep up with its closest competitor, which is providing its workers with less personal insurance coverage, higher deductibles, and no family coverage. The pressure on Alliance to downgrade its coverage is strong. Mark Held, president of Alliance, has resisted that pressure, with the firm belief that providing good coverage is the right thing to do. As he says: "If we switched to their plan, we'd save $3 million a year. The solution is a national health plan that would spread the cost of insurance evenly across the largest pool possible. A single-payer plan would accomplish this, and level the playing field."[63]*

Hospitals, nursing homes, and other facilities will win by having their funding stabilized through predictable global budgets. Many facilities, especially those in underserved areas, will be able to stay and contribute to their communities. As long as facilities can demonstrate their need in community service, they will find a more stable environment than they now have.

Most physicians and other health professionals will also do well under NHI. Those in shortage fields can expect more stable and higher reimbursement. All patients will be insured and "paying patients". Providers will have much less bureaucracy to deal with, together with more clinical autonomy. Second-guessing by faceless clerks in the employ of multiple payers and health plans will be a thing of the past, replaced by simplified billing procedures and clarified coverage and reimbursement policies.

Government, at both state and federal levels, also joins the winners' circle with NHI. It gains an opportunity to build a more accountable health care delivery system that offers better health outcomes at lower costs. It will see a higher return on its investments in health care, and be in a better position to contain health care spending, improve the population's health, and increase economic productivity. At the same time, NHI can help to strengthen our social solidarity and restore the public's faith in responsible government.

There will be losers, to be sure, with NHI. These include the private insurance industry, which will be banned from offering coverage that is duplicative to that of the public program. Other stakeholders in the medical industrial complex, such as the drug and medical device industries, which for many years have been able to set their own prices, will find their profits brought under public scrutiny and constrained. They will still be able to earn reasonable profits if they compete well in providing safe and cost-effective products that benefit patients. And if they succeed, their potential markets will be large. Others who will be constrained by NHI include those physicians and other health care professionals who are now receiving more reimbursement than they have earned by providing inappropriate and unnecessary services.

## The Decision Before Us

Deciding between multi-payer and single-payer health care financing is not a close call. It should be obvious by now that we need fundamental change in the way we finance health care in this country. Boiled down to the essence of reform, the main choice is between retaining a multi-payer system, as we have now, or moving to single-payer NHI. As more and more Americans fare worse under today's system, including so many battling against cancer, the stakes get higher every day.

All the evidence over many years shows that single-payer, despite stakeholder rhetoric and disinformation to the contrary, is a more efficient and fiscally responsible way to finance universal coverage with improved access, quality and equity. It will meet all four of the American Cancer Society's 4 As, whereas multi-payer is 0 for 4.

Paul Krugman, Ph.D., Professor of Economics at Princeton University and the 2008 Nobel laureate in Economics, has this to say on the matter:

"Good economics is also good politics: reformers will do best with a straight forward single-payer plan, which offers maximum savings and, unlike the Clinton plan, can easily be explained. We need to do this one right. If reform fails again, we'll be on the way to a radically unequal society, in which all but the most affluent Americans face the constant risk of financial ruin and even premature death because they can't pay their medical bills."[64]

# References:

1. Press Release. American Cancer Society launches nationwide awareness campaign to spotlight challenges to the U.S. health care system. Atlanta, GA. American Cancer Society, September 17, 2007.
2. Ibid # 1.
3. Wender RC. The adequacy of the access-to-care debate: Looking through the cancer lens. *CANCER* 110 (2): 232, 2007.
4. Reeder CE, Gordon D. Managing oncology costs. *Am J Manag Care* 12 (suppl): S 3-S19, 2006.
5. McKoy JM, Fitzner KA, Edwards BJ, et al. Cost considerations in the management of cancer in the older patient. *Oncology* 21 (7): 851-60, 2007.
6. Bach PB. Costs of cancer care: a view from the Centers for Medicare & Medicaid Services. *J Clin Oncol* 25 (2): 187-90, 2007.
7. Hewitt M, Greenfield S, Stovall E, eds. *From Cancer Patient to Cancer Survivor: Lost in Transition.* Washington, D.C. The National Academies Press, 2006, p 31.
8. McQueen MP. The shifting calculus of workplace benefits. *Wall Street Journal,* January 16, 2007: D 1.
9. Goodman A. Study reveals gaps in insurance coverage for adult survivors of

cancer. *Oncology Times,* March 25, 2006, p 24

10. Geyman JP. *Do Not Resuscitate: Why the Health Insurance Industry Is Dying, and How We Must Replace It*. Monroe, ME. Common Courage Press, 2008, pp 92-111.

11. Ibid # 10, p 113.

12. New York State Department of Insurance. Consumer Guide to HMOs. Choices available for individual coverage. Accessed on April 28, 2009 at http://www.ins. state.ny.us/consumer/cg hmo2008.pdf.

13. New York State Department of Insurance. Premium rates for standard individual health plans. New York County. Accessed on April 28, 2009 at http://www.ins. state.ny.us/hmorates/html/hmonewyo.htm.

14. The Public and the Health Care Delivery System. Summary & Chartpack. NPR/ Kaiser Family Foundation/Harvard School of Public Health, April 2009.

15. Haynes VD. The health-care punch: Insurance costs are a blow even when employers cover more of the tab. , February 2-8, 2009, p 7.

16. Sinibaldi J. A broker's lament: We brought this on ourselves. The Health Care Blog, March 9, 2009. Accessed at http://www.thehealthcareblog.com/the_ health_care_blog/2009/03/a...

17. Ibid # 10, pp 123-54.

18. AHIP Press release. AHIP announces proposal to expand access to health insurance coverage to every American. Washington, D.C., November 13, 2006.

19. America's Health Insurance Plans (AHIP). Guaranteeing access to coverage for all Americans, December 19, 2007.

20. Angell M. Health reform you shouldn't believe in. *The American Prospect* April 21, 2008.

21. Kaiser Family Foundation. Headed for a Crunch: An Update on Medicaid Spending, Coverage and Policy Heading into an Economic Downturn. September, 2008.

22. Sack, K. Recession drove many to Medicaid last year. *New York Times*, October 1, 2010: A16.

23. Johnson K, Abelson R. Model in Utah may be future for Medicaid. *New York Times*, February 24, 2005.

24. Solomon D. Wrestling with Medicaid cuts. *Wall Street Journal,* February 16, 2006: A4.

25. Centers for Medicare and Medicaid Services (CMS). CMS proposes new rules for redesigning Medicaid; states have greater flexibility in benefits, cost-sharing. February 21, 2008.

26. Bishop H, Clark P, Leopold B, et al. 2007 CCH Medicare and Medicaid Benefits. Chicago, IL: Wolters Kluwer, 2007.

27. Lung Cancer Connections. Caring 4Cancer. An introduction to Medicaid. Web site accessed October 31, 2008.

28. Ward E, Halpern M, Schrag N. et al. Association of insurance with cancer care utilization and outcomes. *CA Cancer J Clin* 58: 9-31, 2008.

29. Anderson GF. From 'soak the rich' to 'soak the poor': recent trends in hospital pricing. *Health Aff (Millwood)* 26: 780-89, 2007.

30. Banthin JS, Bernard DM. Changes in financial burdens for health care: national estimates for the population younger than 65 years, 1996 to 2003. *JAMA* 296: 2712-19, 2006.

31. Himmelstein DU, Warren E, Thorne D, et al. Illness and injury as contributors to bankruptcy. *Health Aff (Millwood)* (suppl) W5-63-W65-73, 2005.

32. Ibid # 28, p 30.

33. Whittington E, ed. Insurance for clinical trial care a state-by-state battle. *CURE* Spring, 2008, pp 14, 53.

34. Oklahoma State Senate. Press release. Senate passes 'Steffanie's Law' amendment. April 17, 2008.

35. Ibid # 5.

36. Talarico, G, Chen, G, Pazdur R. Enrollment of elderly patients in clinical trials for cancer drug registration: a 7-year experience by the US Food and Drug Administration. *J Clin Oncol* 22: 4626-31, 2004.

37. Wolfe SM. The uninsured in the United States: what the drop to 45.7 million means. *Health Letter* 24 (11): 2, 2008.

38. Evans RG. Separate and unequal: self-segregation in health insurance. *Medical Care* 46 (10): 1014, 2008.

39. Medicare Rights Center. Medical record. New York. *Asclepios* 8 (43), October 23, 2008.

40. Woolhandler S, Campbell T, Himmelstein DU. Costs of health care administration in the United States and Canada. *N Engl J Med* 349: 768, 2003.

41. Fronstein P. Annual Claims Distribution "20/80 Rule". Outlook on consumerism in health care. EBRI. Washington, DC. Employee Benefit Research Institute.

42. Krugman P. The world of U.S. health care economics is downright scary. *Seattle Post-Intelligencer*, September 26, 2006: B1.

42. Himmelstein DU. The National Health Program Slide-show Guide, Center for National Health Program Studies. Cambridge, MA, 2000.

44. Kahn JG, Kronick R, Kreger M, et al. The cost of health insurance in California: Estimates for insurers, physicians, and hospitals. *Health Aff (Millwood)* 24 (6): 1-11, 2005.

45. Kagel R. Blue crossroads: Insurance in the 21st Century. *American Medical News,* September 20, 2004.

46. Grembowski DE, Diehr P, Novak LC, et al. Measuring the "managedness" and covered benefits of health plans. *Health Service Research* 35 (3): 707, 2000.

47. Ibid # 40, updated to 2008 dollars.

48. Geyman JP. S*hredding the Social Contract: The Privatization of Medicare.* Monroe, ME. Common Courage Press, 2008, pp131-37.

49. Fisher ES, Welch HG. Avoiding the unintended consequences of growth in medical care: how might more be worse? *JAMA* 281: 446-53. 1999.

50. Wennberg JB, Fisher ES, Skinner JS. Geography and the debate over Medicare reform. *Health Affairs Web Exclusive* W-103, February 13, 2002.

51. Boccuti C, Moon M. Comparing Medicare and private insurers: growth rates in spending over three decades. *Health Aff (Millwood)* 22 (2): 235, 2003.

52. Woolhandler S, Himmelstein DU. The National Health Program Slideshow Guide, Cambridge, MA. Center for National Health Program Studies, 2000.

53. Lu JFR, Hsiao WC. Does universal health insurance make health care unaffordable? Lessons from Taiwan. *Health Aff (Millwood)* 22 (3): 77-88, 2003, as updated by Cheng TM in a presentation to the annual meeting of Physicians for a National Health Program, San Diego, CA, October 25, 2008.

54. Kuttner R. Market-based failure – a second opinion on U.S. health care costs. *N Engl J Med* 358 (6): 549-51, 2008.

55. Woolhandler S, Himmelstein DU. Paying for national health insurance – and not getting it. *Health Aff (Millwood)* 21 (4): 88-98, 2002.

56. Gross D. National health care? We're halfway there. *New York Times*, December 3, 2006.

57. Woolhandler S. Interview. Unhealthy solutions: Private insurance, high cost and the denial of care. *Multinational Monitor* September/October, 2008, p 38.

58. Carrasquillo O, Himmelstein DU, Woolhandler S. A reappraisal of private employers' role in providing health insurance. *N Engl J Med* 340 (2): 109-14, 1999.

59. Harrison JA. Paying more, getting less. *Dollars & Sense.* May/June 2008.

60. Ibid #10, p 187.

61. GM Inside News & GM Forum. Leveling the playing field. Detroit, MI. August 22, 2005.

62. Zakaria F. Worthwhile Canadian initiative. *Newsweek*, February 7, 2009.

63. Bard R. Benefit to business: Executive says single-payer is the solution. Health Care for All-Washington, January-March, 2009, p 1.

64. Krugman P. One nation, uninsured. *New York Times,* June 13, 2005.

CHAPTER 10

# Myths and Lies as Barriers to Health Care Reform

"You can fool all the people some of the time, and some of the people all the time, but you cannot fool all the people all the time."[1]

—Abraham Lincoln

"I believe we've been told a story about America that simply isn't true. But we've been told it so often that it seems true. It's a story of no possibility – of too few resources and no political will; of fear and lack of compassion; of individual consumerist values at home and 'America only' policies abroad. But Americans are better than the current story says we are, and Americans have begun to question this story. Now we need a new story about who we are and what we might do together as a country."[2]

—Former U.S. Senator Bill Bradley
All-American and professional basketball player,
three-term New Jersey Senator and author of *The New American Story*

In the midst of our current economic crisis, skepticism that markets are always best and receptivity to regulation aimed at delivering important social values are both rising fast. The ideas we have been sold on health care reform are stale, worn out and broken – and most everyone recognizes this.

When it comes to health care reform, we have been sold a bill of goods by those who ardently believe that the best way to deliver health care is through a market-based system. As we have seen in cancer care, profit motives all too often trump service, as patients and their families struggle as much against the system as against their disease. But if we are ever going to be able to resolve our increasing system problems of access, costs, quality and equity, we must challenge the myths and lies in order to control the debate over health care reform.

The first step in dealing with them is to understand them.

Myths, lies and disinformation distort the real issues of health care and distract us from effective approaches to reform. To the extent that they carry the day, they block meaningful reform, as they already have for many years. As such, these myths are a serious challenge to our democracy and the public interest, since without reform our system continues to deteriorate, leaving growing millions of Americans without access to care for such serious diseases as cancer. In his commencement address at Yale University in June 1962, the late President John F. Kennedy had this to say on the subject:

"For the great enemy of truth is very often not the lie – deliberate, contrived and dishonest – but the myth – persistent, persuasive, and unrealistic. Too often we hold fast to the clichés of our forebears. We subject all facts to a prefabricated set of interpretations. We enjoy the comfort of opinion without the discomfort of thought."[3]

The facts are clear about problems of our health care system – from this book and previous books of mine as well as many others. Yet those opposed to single-payer and other reforms of unfettered markets are good at never letting the facts get in the way of their argument to maintain the status quo. What ploys, half-truths and lies need to be exposed so the facts can dominate the debate?

Obfuscation of the health care debate can be boiled down to twelve falsehoods that are trotted out before the public whenever another round of reform threatens the marketplace (Table 10.1). The first six are of more general nature, the last six relate to scare tactics deployed by market advocates against single-payer national health insurance (NHI).

## Myths Versus Reality

Abraham Lincoln noted the century-old power of deceptive words in our early history. And as Bill Bradley reminds us above, myths often become repeated so often as to become part of our culture and language. As expected, market stakeholders and their allies often promulgate these

TABLE 10.1

# TWELVE COMMON MYTHS ABOUT U.S. HEALTH CARE

1. The free market can bring its "greater efficiency" to bear in solving health care system problems.
2. Multi-payer financing offers increased choice, not "one size fits all."
3. We have the best health care system in the world.
4. Incremental reform of health care will work better than radical reform.
5. We don't, and shouldn't, ration care in this country.
6. Our health care financing is mostly private.
7. NHI would be socialized medicine.
8. NHI will lead to excess bureaucracy.
9. NHI will stifle innovation.
10. Patients will over-utilize NHI and break the bank.
11. NHI will lead to excessive wait times, as in other single-payer countries.
12. NHI will raise my taxes.

myths in an effort to perpetuate the status quo and avoid regulation and accountability. But unless these myths are examined and tested against evidence, they can cloud our vision and limit our capacity to solve problems. Here are the twelve most important myths that can readily be discredited by the facts:

**1. The free market can bring its "greater efficiency" to bear in solving health care system problems.**

The conservative Dallas-based think tank, the National Center for Policy Analysis, makes one of the best cases for this view:

"Single-payer health insurance differs from many private insurance companies in one important respect—no profit motive. But, far from [stockholders] being a burden, having no stockholders removes any incentive to operate efficiently. In fact, national health insurance provides all the wrong incentives for both the health care system itself and the patients in the system."[4]

This is typical boilerplate for the alleged myth of market efficiency, as it may work in other sectors of the economy. In Chapter 6, however, we have already seen many ways in which a deregulated marketplace in health care increases costs, decreases access, and often compromises the quality of care. Recall some of the ways – more consolidation than competition in the marketplace, wide latitude of providers and suppliers to set prices at what the traffic will bear, and overuse of services (often inappropriate or unnecessary) through *physician-induced demand.*

There are many other examples that discredit the ability of markets to fix health care system problems. Private Medicare plans would be bankrupt if forced to compete with traditional Medicare on a level playing field. What saves them are heavy subsidies from the government. Consider the evidence, as these reports indicate:

- Medicare+Choice HMOs were subsidized by overpayments that averaged 13 percent between 1998 and 2000. Yet despite this assistance, many still left the market because the profits were insufficient. This exodus left 2.4 million seniors to find alternate coverage and often other physicians.[5]
- The General Accounting Office (GAO) and Congressional Budget Office (CBO) have both concluded that private Medicare plans are less efficient and more expensive than traditional Medicare, and by no small margin. They concluded that the difference is actually to the point of threatening the long-term fiscal sustainability of Medicare.[6,7]
- A 2008 report by the GAO looked at enrollees in private Medicare plans. It found that more than one-half of those 8 million enrollees had no annual limits on out-of-pocket spending for serious medical problems, thereby offering no protection against catastrophic medical bills. In contrast, traditional Medicare does cap out-of-pocket spending.[8]
- Based on his research, MIT economist Jonathan Gruber has concluded that tax policies which fund expanded public coverage are much more efficient than those that fund private health insurance.[9]

If competition were becoming more intense so that the consumer was better served, markets for health insurance would be expanding. Instead, private markets for health insurance are *shrinking* as their costs go up and coverage goes down. Public markets in private Medicare and Medicaid plans are also threatened as a backlash to government subsidies builds in hard economic times. The only greater efficiency that private health insurance has over public financing is in denial management, a rapidly growing industry in itself, whose aim is to manage patient and physician dissatisfaction with what the insurance company is refusing to cover.[10]

Private insurers hold fast to the "20/80" rule as they pursue the 80 percent of Americans who are healthiest and have the lowest medical costs, leaving the sicker 20 percent of the population who need insurance the most to be uninsured or in search of public coverage (Figure 10.1). That basic orientation, insure the healthy and flee the sick, is perhaps one of the most telling pieces of evidence against the

## FIGURE 10.1

## Annual Claims Distribution: The "20/80 Rule"

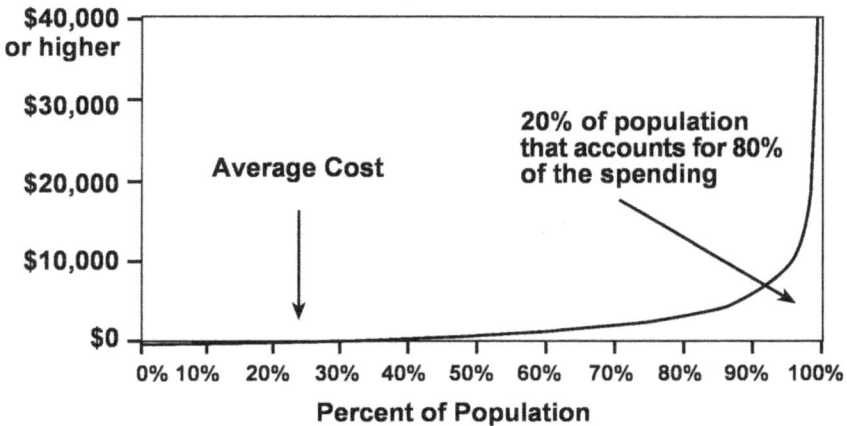

Source: Fronstin P. Outlook on Consumerism in Health Care. Washington, D.C. Employee Benefit Research Institute (EBRI), 2008, p.9. Reprinted with permission.

claim that markets for health insurance better serve the consumer.[11]

Behind the myths, even the insurance industry itself is starting to admit that it has proven itself too expensive, too unreliable, and too inefficient to sustain itself, never mind bring efficiencies to the system.

It knows it is pricing itself out of existence, and its future is limited. Mike Bartlett is executive vice president and chief financial officer of BlueCross BlueShield of Michigan (BCBSM), one of the remaining not-for-profit BCBS plans in the country. The plan is now reporting uncontrollable financial losses that threaten its future viability. It is making an appeal to the Attorney General of Michigan for increased state regulations to prevent other carriers from dumping higher-risk individuals on BCBS as a last-resort private carrier. Bartlett paints his company's plight in stark terms:

> "Michigan's individual health insurance market is set up to fail financially. It's a hard truth, especially if you oppose reforming the market, but it is the truth."[12]

The industry has deteriorated to the point where Wall Street has begun to realize it is financially sick. Like most stocks in 2008, the share values of the top 5 insurers fell sharply. But unlike the S & P 500's drop of 38 percent, the leading health insurers fell by 50 to 70 percent (Table 10.2).[13] An October 2008 article in the *Wall Street Journal* expressed concern over how the industry will navigate a worsening economy, increasing unemployment, and the impact of declining tax revenues on public programs.[14] In the fourth week of February 2009, reacting to the news of impending reimbursement cuts for private Medicare plans, the stock of Humana, the second largest provider of Medicare Advantage plans, plummeted by 24 percent in a selloff.[15] And by the end of the week, the stock values of the Big Five insurers plunged as shown in Figure 10.2.[16]

Some private insurers are also seeing the writing on the wall, and are moving into the money-managing business by opening their own banks, especially to manage tax-sheltered health savings accounts. UnitedHealth and Blue Cross have chartered their own banks and set up special credit cards to manage HSAs, now an industry of its own with some $1 billion in annual fees.[17]

In light of the industry teetering on the brink, searching for and getting government handouts, and resorting to creating new businesses like banks in a desperate attempt to survive, the suggestion that private enterprise brings "efficiency" to health insurance is at best a cruel joke, and at worst a lucrative enterprise for lobbyists and a few well-paid upper managers.

# TABLE 10.2

## BIG 5 HEALTH INSURANCE INDUSTRY PLAYERS, 2008

| Ticker | Company | Market Cap | Employees | Stock Drop YTD | Share Price 12/31/08 |
|---|---|---|---|---|---|
| UNH | United HealthCare | $32 B | $67,000 | 52% | $26.00 |
| WLP | Wellpoint Anthem | $21 B | $42,000 | 51% | $42.13 |
| AET | Aetna | $13 B | $35,000 | 50% | $28.50 |
| CI | Cigna | $5 B | $27,000 | 70% | $16.85 |
| HUM | Humana | $6 B | $27,000 | 52% | $37.28 |
|  | S&P 500 |  |  | 38% |  |

$90 Billion in Lost Value for 5 Companies in 2008

Source: Personal communication, Rob Stone, M.D., January 20, 2009.

## 2. Multi-payer financing is superior because it offers increased choice, instead of single-payer's "one size fits all."

America's Health Insurance Plans (AHIP), the industry's trade group representing 1,300 private insurers, spells out a wonderful mission to "expand access to high quality, cost effective health care to all Americans, and to ensure Americans' financial security through robust insurance markets, product flexibility and innovation, and an abundance of consumer choice."[18] However, there is a gaping gap between that stated mission and the reality they pursue. First, private insurance no longer provides many enrollees much security against catastrophic costs of health care, which after all, is what most of us are looking for in insurance; and second, many supposed "choices" are not really choices at all. Five examples illustrate these points:

FIGURE 10.2

## Big 5 Health Insurers
## Share Performance for Week of
## February 23-27, 2009

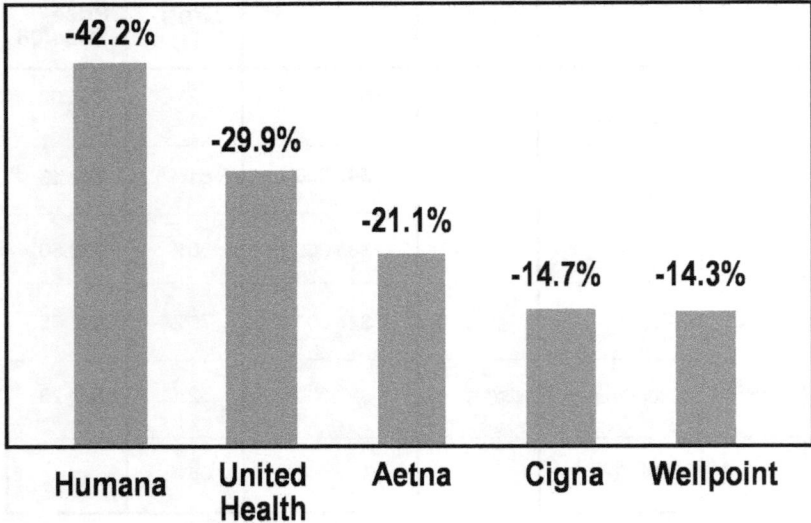

Source: Jannarone J. Health care gets a shock treatment. *Wall Street Journal*,
February, 27, 2009: C 10.

• There are many circumstances under which enrollees have
no choice. A sacred choice, frequently trumpeted by advocates
of the status quo, is the right to choose one's doctor. But when
insurers make changes in a network's providers and hospitals,
add new restrictions in fine print, and use lock-in rules to prevent people from changing plans when they want or need to, this
choice disappears. These hurdles do not exist in a single-payer
system when patients have full choice of providers.
• Two of the largest employers in the country, Wal-Mart and
McDonalds, offer health insurance to their employees, making
their businesses important symbols for how health insurance
works in America, and in this case how choice works. If a
worker at Wal-Mart or McDonalds can only afford a limited

benefit policy with an annual cap on coverage of $1,000 to $2,500 (meaning the insurer pays for a maximum of $2,500 in medical care, hardly enough to cover even a broken arm let alone care for a complicated disease like cancer), it becomes clear to everyone that the policy is not about choice, or even about health care. The primary benefit of such a policy is a PR ploy for the employer; Wal-Mart and McDonalds can say "we offer health insurance," confident that the details of what is essentially a sham won't dent the public relations benefit.[19] By contrast, Wal-Mart and McDonald's both operate in Canada, where they don't have to offer insurance because every employee is fully covered by their single-payer system.

- "Choice" is axiomatically a good idea – everyone is behind it. And because private enterprise is equated with broad choice, such as the breadth experienced on, say, a supermarket shelf, it is a small leap to believe that private insurance provides choice. But a 2005 study by the Commonwealth Fund found that only 53 percent of working adults under 65 are offered two or more choices of health plans by their employer. Choice is often thought of as a matter of personal preference. But that same study found another factor at work, income: lower-income workers have the least choice.[20] In a single-payer system, choice is not mediated by income, and everyone has the same amount of choice.

- Choice in the marketplace, as everyone understands, is a function of competition: the more businesses competing to deliver a service, the more choice the consumer has. Yet a study by the American Medical Association has found near-monopolies by private insurers in 95 percent of HMO/PPO markets covering 43 states.[21] As even the most ardent free-market theorist can attest, monopolies and choice don't mix. Opponents of single-payer point out, correctly, that NHI is itself a monopoly system. But there are important distinctions. First, the consumer is not victimized by price gouging because patients don't pay out-of-pocket. Second, monopoly pressure is indeed exerted, as every opponent of single-payer points out, on drug company pricing. This is the effect of a monopoly, but it is one in the service of the patient and the taxpayer, who are one and the same.

- These monopolies of the health insurance market extend in many directions. For example, just three large insurers together hold a market share more than 65 percent in 32 percent of states, as previously shown in Figure 8.1.[22] Such conditions not only inhibit choice but foster other problems such as price-fixing as well.

## 3. We have the best health care system in the world.

As discussed at length in Chapter 6, a widespread myth lives on that we have the best health care system in the world, despite an enormous literature to the contrary. This belief seems to be driven by our comparative wealth, abundance of technology, and high level of specialization. It is also fueled by corporations and investors who profit from our continuing to waste more money on overhead and profits than most countries spend delivering health care. But when we look at the evidence, we have the opportunity to lift the veil of arrogant American exceptionalism that insists we are the best. And when we drop our insistence that we must be the leader, we are then free to incorporate the best ideas of other countries as well as our own.

We offered some evidence in Chapter 6 countering claims that U.S. cancer care is the best in the world. Destroying this myth is essential if we are to achieve single-payer. As long as we are led to believe we are Number One, our efforts to fight the war on cancer are neatly constrained within the box of our current system. To that end, here is additional evidence to the contrary for both overall health care and cancer care.

- This just in: we are *last!* The latest National Scorecard on U.S. Health System Performance, as reported by the Commonwealth Fund, shows that this country fell from 15th among 19 countries to last between 2006 and 2008 on a measure of mortality that is amenable to medical care (Figure 10.3); it is estimated that 101,000 fewer Americans would die prematurely each year if this country could achieve the lower mortality rates of the leading countries.[23]

FIGURE 10.3

## Percentage Decline in Mortality from Amenable Causes and Other Causes of Death Among Males Ages 0-74 in Nineteen Countries from 1997-98 to 2002-03

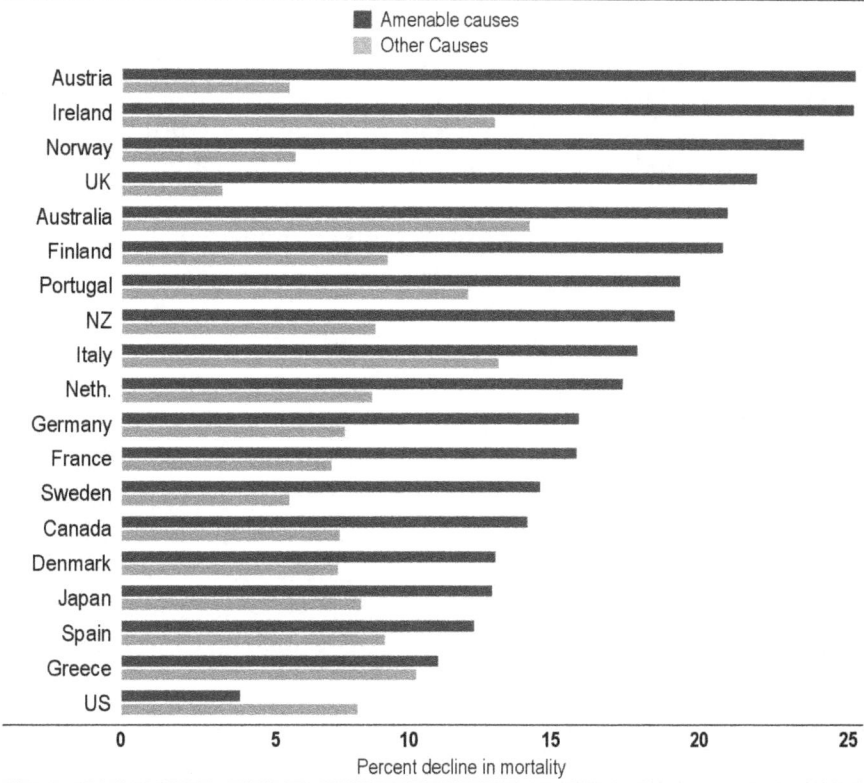

Source: The Commonwealth Fund Commission on a High Performance Health System. *Why Not the Best? Results from the National Scorecard on U.S. Health System Performance.* Vol. 97, July 17, 2008. Reprinted with permission.

- Falling behind "old Europe", a 2007 report ranked the U.S. 42nd in the world for life expectancy, lower than most of Europe and Japan[24]
- Another 2007 study found that Canada has at least the quality of care as this country, often with better outcomes, despite spending little more than one-half what we spend on health care.[25]

- An earlier study demonstrated conclusively that poor women with cancer in Toronto have better outcomes than their counterparts in Detroit, even after accounting for race and standards of measuring poverty (e.g., survival rates more than 50 percent higher for lung, stomach and pancreatic cancer compared to American women in Detroit's poorest districts).[26]
- A 2006 report found that Americans in late middle age are less healthy than their counterparts in England for cancer and five other chronic diseases.[27]
- Having health insurance as well as a source of primary care has been found necessary to achieve quality of care;[28] however, the U.S. has been found to rank last on 11 performance criteria in primary care compared to 11 other industrial countries.[29] Moreover, patients living in regions with larger numbers of specialists compared to primary care physicians are more likely to have late-stage colorectal cancer when first diagnosed.[30]
- As we have already seen in Table 7.1, investor-owned hospitals, HMOs, nursing homes and mental health centers provide more expensive care of lower quality than not-for-profit facilities.[31] For-profit hospices reap profits way above the costs of not-for-profit hospices, typically employing less expensive labor, including fewer registered nurses, medical social workers, and fewer clinicians.[32] Other countries that best us on various quality measures lack these for-profit sectors, suggesting they are part of our problem, not part of the solution.

There is still more evidence that the quality of care in this country leaves much to be desired. As we have seen in earlier chapters, perverse incentives in our market-based system lead many physicians to provide too much care that is inappropriate and unnecessary. Here are just two examples of how excess care adversely affects patients:

- In their ongoing studies of regional variations in U.S. health care, researchers at Dartmouth Medical School have found that seniors living in areas with increased use of technology and specialist services have worse outcomes.[33]
- Another study by the Dartmouth research group found that patients living in higher-spending areas of the country, as

compared to their counterparts living in lower-spending areas, have higher mortality over a five-year period after experiencing heart attack, hip fracture, or diagnosis of colorectal cancer.[34]

All of this has led Dr. Barbara Starfield, Professor of Health Policy and Management at the Johns Hopkins Bloomberg School of Public Health, to this observation:

"It is high time that U.S. health services researchers broaden their efforts to address current issues of who should provide what and to what level of performance. Thirty years of Dartmouth studies showing great overuse of specialty services have not resulted in questioning the increasing specialty orientation of the health services system or devoting attention to the quality of specialty care."[35]

4. **Incremental reform of health care will work better than radical reform, and more fundamental reform is not politically feasible.**

This view is shared by many, including of course all of the stakeholders in our multi-payer system, their allies, investors in new incremental "reforms" (such as HSAs, disease management, and information management industries), and many others who either deny or are unaware of the long record of failure of any incremental efforts to manage our system problems of access, cost, quality and equity.

The battlefield of health policy is littered with the debris of many failed incremental plans, no matter how much fanfare and hope they generated when first introduced. If we can learn from over 30 years of experience, the main lesson is that none have been effective. In effect, all of these incremental "reforms" have served market advocates and the private insurance industry well by perpetuating our deregulated system and avoiding their accountability for our worsening problems. Market stakeholders have so far won a victory through the ineffectiveness of these "reforms", which make it appear that the system is so complicated that no reform can work. This ramping down of expectations is a huge boon to advocates of the status quo.

A look at a list of some of the attempted "reforms" and why they have all failed or will fail is instructive. Understanding some of these various ruses will make it easier to cut through the confusion generated by new ones that inevitably get churned out.

- **Consumer-Directed Health Care (CDHC).** Managed care of the 1980s and 1990s failed to contain health care costs while adding greatly to the complexity and bureaucracy of the health care marketplace. Its sequel, CDHC, shares qualities with grade B movie sequels: we get caught up in the hope they do it better this time but, of course, they always disappoint. CDHC still fails to contain costs or to expand comprehensive coverage. Robert Evans, Ph.D., the well-known health economist at the University of British Columbia mentioned earlier, has this to say about the CDHC effort:

    "In the United States, financing gimmicks (i.e. Health Savings Accounts, Consumer-Directed Health Care) provide cover stories for policies that, whatever else they may do, will inevitably transfer costs back from taxpayers to users of care, from the healthy and wealthy to the unhealthy and unwealthy, without any threat to providers' incomes."[36]

- **Mandates.** Whether requiring employers to cover all their workers or requiring all individuals to purchase insurance (with governmental subsidies for those with sufficiently low income), mandates may seem from the headlines to be a new 21st century wrinkle worth trying. But all have failed for three decades to provide universal coverage of adequate insurance. Not for lack of trying, however: Hawaii in 1974; Massachusetts in 1988; Oregon in 1989; Tennessee and Minnesota in 1992; Washington in 1993; Maine in 2003; and Massachusetts again in 2006. The story is always the same: persistent levels of about 10 to 15 percent uninsured, many underinsured, increased bureaucratic costs and waste, and no effective cost containment.[37]

    The latest highly touted "Massachusetts Miracle" mandate of 2006 is revealing when stacked up against the ideological arguments for free markets, deregulation, efficiency and consumer choice that the proponents of multi-payer are extolling. One aspect of the Massachusetts mandate gives a new meaning to the concept of consumer choice: it forces people to buy insurance from private companies. If consumers choose not to buy, they face fines of $1,000. Another aspect of the "miracle" is its impact on cost control: the cost of governmental subsidies to the insurance companies are much higher than expected. Costs remain high enough that many enrollees still forego necessary care due to costs. Finally, despite the added costs, despite the fines, the program still fails to cover everyone. Three years after the program was enacted, these are the real results:[38]

- Although about one-half of the previously uninsured now have some coverage, universal coverage was not, and will not be achieved.
- Many lower-income people who previously had care under the State's old free-care program now face cost-sharing that leads many to forego needed care.
- The once high administrative overhead of the private plans now have an added layer of 4 to 5 percent for the public "Connector" established by the law to implement the program.
- The program has cost much more than anticipated: $1.3 billion in fiscal 2009; Massachusetts now spends 33% more per person for health care than the national per capita average.[39]
- During the state's budget crisis in the Fall of 2008, Governor Deval Patrick, in order to keep the program going, was forced to make budget cuts in safety net programs, including providers, Emergency Rooms, primary care, and chronic mental health services.

Compare those predictable outcomes with a statewide single-payer program, which would assure comprehensive coverage for all state residents, while actually saving the state about $8 to $10 billion annually through reduced administrative costs.

- **Information Technology**. Wider application of information technology (IT) is seen by its proponents as an obvious way to improve efficiency of our system and even save costs. IT is part of any reform package now under consideration, and many policy makers see it as a silver bullet for system problems. A new federal Office of the National Health Information Technology Coordinator was established in 2004 with the hope that it could save health care costs by up to 20 percent a year.[40] Investors and vendors have been attracted to potentially lucrative new markets for the further development of electronic medical records (EMRs) and various Web-based resources. But while there is no question that EMRs greatly improve communication and efficiency in many medical practices and that Internet access can help patients find information useful to their seeking care, there are many reasons why IT cannot be expected to reform the larger system. What have we gained, for example, by improving communication between physicians and the 17,000 health plans in Chicago?! The cost of IT equipment is high, and there is no consensus within the health care establishment about the most useful ways to adopt IT. Plans and performance objectives have yet to be developed, and there is limited trust between physicians, insurers, and digital record-keepers. More than 40 percent of federal contractors and state Medicaid agencies using EMRs have experienced privacy breaches of personal health information.[41,42] Moreover, there is no evidence that IT can contain costs at all, and may even lead to increased costs.[43,44]

- **Chronic Disease Management**. Since chronic illness accounts for almost 75 percent of annual health care expenditures, it is a logical target for cost containment efforts.[45] The concept is that better communication and team care of chronic illness can improve quality of care and perhaps save money. Effective programs have been developed and have been operational for some years by primary care teams in non-for-profit HMOs such as Group Health Cooperative and Kaiser Permanente. But a whole new "disease management" (DM) industry has burgeoned since the 1990s that just adds another layer of bureaucracy and mostly bypasses primary care. Introduced by the drug industry, a for-profit commercial DM industry has emerged that attempts to provide patient education and improved self-management of chronic diseases. Nurses in distant call centers call patients at regular intervals with reminders and advice, often without involvement of the patient's own physician. The original idea for drug companies, of course, was that this approach could lead to increased use of its own products. But the verdict on costs is in: The CBO has already concluded that disease management will *not* reduce overall health care spending.[46] And a recent RAND analysis of 317 studies drew the same conclusion, adding also that "payers and policy makers should remain skeptical about vendor claims and should demand supporting evidence based on transparent and scientifically sound methods."[47]

• **High-Risk Pools.** Some 30 states have established high-risk pools, favored by private insurers and supported by state and federal funding, in an attempt to extend insurance coverage to those who have been denied coverage in the individual market. But this approach has been expensive and has failed on many counts. It has small impact (covers only 180,000 people nationwide), high premiums, limited benefits, extended waiting lists, and limited state and federal budgets.[48]

• **Association Health Plans (AHPs).** This approach, also touted by the private insurance industry, serves their interest more than their enrollees. These are plans that allow private insurers to better market their policies across state lines. Insurers claim that AHPs can make insurance more affordable for smaller employers. But instead, AHPs give them an opportunity to seek out the least regulated states, avoid rate-setting regulations, and cherry pick the market without assurances of adequate coverage. The CBO has found that AHPs fail to contain costs, and that most small employers end up paying more.[49] A 2005 report by Families USA that looked into AHPs identified widespread evidence of bait and switch premium hikes, excessive cost-sharing, misrepresentation of benefits, and other examples of fraud and abuse.[50]

As described more fully elsewhere,[51] all these incremental tweaks around the margins of our system fail for six main reasons:

1. They disregard history and previous failures.
2. They address the wrong targets (e.g., privatizing Medicare to "address" the high costs of prescription drugs instead of negotiating discounted prices).
3. They assume that markets can fix our problems.
4. Market stakeholders hijack and exploit attempted reforms (e.g. the 2003 Medicare legislation).

5. Patchwork approaches don't deal with the many perverse incentives throughout the system.
6. Most importantly, they prop up and retain an obsolete private insurance industry.

We are still being told by moderates and centrists that more incremental "reforms" are the only politically feasible way to proceed. But we know that public financing through single-payer, coupled with a private delivery system transitioned to a not-for-profit basis, will work by redistributing resources, reducing waste, adding efficiency and accountability, increasing access and containing costs. Drawing an analogy with medical care, Dr. David Himmelstein notes "It is unethical to prescribe a placebo when effective therapy is available."[52]

## 5. We don't, and shouldn't, ration care in this country.

This myth is commonly voiced by opponents of single-payer NHI with the assumption that we don't ration care in today's system and that NHI would ration care to our detriment. Both views are incorrect. We already ration care by class and ability to pay, though many deny it. Managed care and its sequel, CDHC, both erect financial barriers to care that exclude many sick people from necessary care. This situation has become dire for much of the population. According to the 2008 Milliman Medical Index, the total cost of medical care for a typical family of four in 2008 was more than $15,600.[53] That means that one-quarter of family income is spent on medical care, much too high a burden to be carried without cutting back on essential care, having worse outcomes and building up large debts.

All payers, whether private or public, must have some cost containment mechanisms available in order to have a viable system. The question is not whether to ration – a necessity in any system – but how, and with what impacts on people? As with any other public payer, NHI will ration – but on the basis of medical need rather than ability to pay. Ineffective services will not be covered, and coverage decisions will be made based on clinical evidence, not whether providers can profit from inappropriate or unnecessary care. Robert Evans weighs in on this issue:

"Universal, compulsory, tax-financed health care systems base access to care on need, not ability to pay, while imposing the cost burden in proportion to tax liability. This benefits the unhealthy and unwealthy at the expense of the healthy and wealthy. Such systems also have access to more effective cost control mechanisms than are available in private markets. The exceptional American reliance on private insurance lies at the root of both exceptional cost escalation and exceptional inequity."[54]

## 6. Our health care financing is mostly private, and that's what makes it work so well.

This myth implies that private financing is better, offers more choice, value, and is better matched to personal needs. By now, you know the mantra. The extent of this myth is suggested by the oft-repeated statement by seniors opposed to publicly-financed NHI that goes along the lines of *"keep the government's hands off my Medicare."*! As earlier chapters have shown, however, the government isn't the enemy, and it serves market stakeholders well to have people believe that. Instead the private insurance industry cherry picks the healthy from the sick and through many deceptive practices takes in at least 20 percent of revenue income in administrative costs and profit.

We already have a financing system in this country that is predominantly public, as indicated by these findings:

- Private employers cover only 21 percent of total health spending in the U.S.[55]
- According to the federal Agency for Healthcare Research and Quality, the government finances 60 percent of the country's annual health care spending through direct payments as well as tax-free exemptions which total about $340 billion a year ($140 billion for employers who offer employer-sponsored insurance and $200 billion for their covered employees);[56] federal funding for uncompensated care to hospitals for care of the uninsured adds an additional 5 percent, so that the federal share becomes about two-thirds of annual health care spending.[57]
- As we saw in the last chapter, public financing of health care in the U.S. now exceeds total health care spending in all comparison industrial countries around the world , all of which have universal coverage. (Figure 9.5)[58]

## 7. NHI is socialized medicine.

Whenever any expansion of public programs for health care is proposed in this country, conservatives and their free-market allies raise the specter of "socialized medicine". The most recent example is the vocal opposition by Republican legislators and the Bush Administration to expansion of SCHIP as a "foot in the door for socialized medicine". But whatever expansion of publicly-financed health insurance that we adopt, whether for children or our entire population through NHI, we retain a private delivery system. So that is not socialized medicine, which involves government ownership of a health care system.

There may be some aspects of NHI that mirror socialism, as is true any time that a government program displaces private initiative, as it does with road-building, police and fire protection. Yet we don't complain about socialism down at the Fire Department because it is widely accepted that the market cannot provide that service reliably and well.

The real question is – socialism for whom? We already have socialism as represented by subsidies the government hands out to private Medicare plans, now $65 billion worth of overpayments over the last five years. When opponents of single-payer complain about socialism, what they mean is that it is socialism for the wrong group because it benefits patients and their families. "Good socialism" means the taxpayer pays for handouts to business, preferably without any strings attached. Paul Krugman has recently coined the term "lemon socialism" for government bailouts where taxpayers bear the costs if things go wrong, but stockholders and executives get the benefits if things go right.[59]

Socialized medicine means that the government owns and operates a national health system, as in England and Spain. Most European countries, Canada, Australia, New Zealand, Japan and Taiwan have one or another form of publicly-financed social health insurance, coupled with a private delivery system. In this country, Medicare is such a system. Except in the VA system, the government does not own and manage hospitals and medical practices. The same will be the case for NHI.

## 8. NHI will lead to excess bureaucracy.

Any large establishment, public or private, needs a bureaucracy to administer it. But the bureaucracy of the private health insurance industry far exceeds that involved in not-for-profit public financing, as shown by these examples.

- The overhead of Medicare averages 3 percent, compared to about 19 percent for commercial carriers and 26.5 percent for investor-owned Blues.[60]
- Although the private insurance market fell by 1 percent between 2000 and 2005, its workforce grew by one-third.[61]
- A 2005 study found that 22 percent of private health insurance premiums in California are spent on sales, marketing, billing, and other administrative tasks that are unnecessary in a publicly-financed program.[62]
- According to the Chicago-based BlueCross BlueShield Association, there are 17,000 different insurance plan designs in Chicago.[63]
- A 2008 survey by the Medical Society of the State of New York found that 93 percent of the physicians surveyed stated that health insurers have required them to change prescription medications, 90 percent said they have had to change the way they treat patients because of insurers' restrictions, and 78 percent are restricted by insurers from referring patients to the physicians they believed would best treat their patients' needs.[64] Compare that with just one set of policies under a single-payer system.
- A 2011 study found that physicians and administrators in Ontario, Canada spent $22, 205 per physician per year interacting with the Canadian single-payer system, just 27 percent of the $82,975 spent annually by U.S. physicians in dealing with our dysfunctional multi-payer system. [65]

Opponents of single-payer are right in one sense: bureaucracy can be a terrible waste of both resources and time, and it needs to be limited to the essentials. What they have yet to grasp, however, is the extent to which bureaucracy hobbles the present multi-payer system and would be minimized by NHI.

## 9. NHI will stifle innovation.

This myth is circulated particularly by health-related industries, such as the drug and medical device industries that want ready access to our delivery system without much government regulation or oversight. It can be answered in several ways.

- Our two large single-payer systems – Medicare and the VA – hardly stifle innovation or incentives for industry to develop and market their products.
- Many real innovations take place abroad, often in countries with universal coverage systems. As an example, CT scanning was developed in England.
- Most claims of "innovation" are marketing hype of "me-too" products, not scientific breakthroughs. Only 32 drugs approved by the FDA between 2000 and 2004 were judged to be innovative by the FDA's criteria (new compounds that are likely to be improvements over drugs already on the market); of these, only 7 were developed by any of the top 10 U.S. drug companies.[66]
- If anything, we err on the side of bringing too many products to market that are neither innovative nor cost-effective. A 1999 report by the Technology Evaluation Committee of Blue Cross and Blue Shield, for example, found that almost one in three evaluations of drugs, medical devices, or procedures were lacking or uncertain in their effectiveness.[67]
- Despite lower (negotiated) drug prices abroad, a number of other countries spend more on R&D than the U.S. (e.g. Sweden spends more than three times as much on R&D per capita than we do),[68] discover new drugs proportionally with this country, and still manage to profit from drug sales.[69]
- Most of the best and most expensive biomedical research in this country is carried out by the government-funded National Institutes of Health (NIH). This would obviously continue under single-payer NHI.
- Industry typically claims undue credit for research that is initially done by NIH and later shifted to industry with hefty government subsidies. One example is the cancer drug Taxol, the best selling oncology drug ever. NIH paid for most of the clinical trials associated with the FDA's approval of the drug,

and later subsidized the patent holder, Bristol-Myers Squibb, in various ways, including payments by Medicare to the company of almost $700 million for patients' use of the drug between 1994 and 1999.[70]

From these examples, we can see that the claim that NHI would stifle innovation rests on the mistaken view that innovation is all about rugged individual entrepreneurs creating breakthroughs in spite of the government, when in reality, the government has long provided crucial support for fostering innovation.

## 10. Because care is "free" to the patients, they will over-utilize NHI and break the bank.

This pervasive myth assumes that patients' appetite for health care is the main driver of people going to the doctor and rising costs of health care. Indeed, the long-held conventional theory of insurance held by many health economists is based on the same premise (moral hazard), holding that patients have to have enough "skin in the game" to avoid using more care than they really need. If it's free, the reasoning goes, people will see their doctor when they don't really need to. Based on this concept, we have seen continued increases in cost-sharing requirements imposed by both private and public payers. The idea here is by having people pay for some portion of the health care services they use, they will be smarter about what they use. However, we have already seen in this book that the more cost-sharing is increased, the more patients forego timely and necessary care, the later cancer and other serious diseases are diagnosed, and the worse the outcomes. John Nyman, Ph.D., health economist at the University of Minnesota, has recently rebutted this premise by showing that cost-sharing, instead of containing costs, actually leads in many cases to adverse clinical outcomes because in order to save money, people cut back on care they really need.[71,72j] In fact, there is an extensive literature that documents the harms of cost-sharing, as these several examples indicate:

- The 2008 Commonwealth Fund's National Scorecard on U.S. Health System Performance found that 37 percent of all U.S. adults reported going without needed care in 2007 because of cost.[73]

- A 2007 systematic review by RAND and the National Bureau of Economic Research examined the literature between 1985 and 2006. They came to a conclusion, as discussed earlier, that increased cost-sharing is associated with increased ER visits, more hospitalizations, and worse outcomes.[74]
- The Kaiser Commission on Medicaid and the Uninsured has concluded that whatever cost "savings" are achieved by cost-sharing result in limits on necessary care.[75]

Since a large amount of necessary care is now being put off because of costs in our multi-payer system, we can anticipate that utilization of services under NHI will go up in the short run. That will result in earlier and better care for many people who had been foregoing needed care. In the long run, however, we will have a system in place with mechanisms to better monitor and control costs through negotiated fees, bulk purchasing by a single purchaser, and global budgets for hospitals and other facilities. Countries with single-payer systems are more successful in containing costs of health care, as demonstrated by Canada over the last three decades. Instead of over-utilization overwhelming single-payer systems, the removal of financial barriers encourages earlier and appropriate care.[76,77] Ironically, but usually not acknowledged by advocates of private insurance, our multi-payer system has built-in incentives to providers and facilities to provide financially rewarding services that are neither appropriate nor necessary.

Overuse of medical care as a result of perverse incentives is a major problem, but not in the way most proponents of the current system suggest. As we have seen in earlier chapters, there are many financial incentives in the health care marketplace for providing expensive care that is inappropriate and unnecessary. These conflicts of interest are far more costly moral hazards than the mythical worry that consumers will gobble up too much chemotherapy and other treatments out of a voracious appetite for health care.

## 11. NHI will lead to excessive wait times.

This is another timeworn myth perpetuated by opponents of publicly-financed health insurance without regard to countervailing evidence. According to the right-wing National Center for Policy Analysis, "When health care is made free at the point of consumption, rationing by waiting is inevitable."[78]

This unfounded assertion seems especially blatant when one considers that NHI provides access to care without financial barriers that otherwise often increase waiting times (if you can get care at all), that all patients are "paying patients" under NHI, and that care is not free anyway since everyone pays into NHI all their lives whether through payroll or income taxes. Moreover, these kinds of evidence below further belie this myth, and show that waiting lines within our system are a growing problem.

- According to a 2008 report by the Commonwealth Fund, only 46 percent of patients in the U.S. could get a rapid appointment with a physician the same or next day in 2007, considerably worse than five other advanced comparison countries that have one or another form of social insurance (Figure 10.4)[79]

FIGURE 10.4

# Waiting Time to See Doctor When Sick or Need Medical Attention Among Sicker Adults, 2007

Percent of adults who could get an appointment on the same or next day

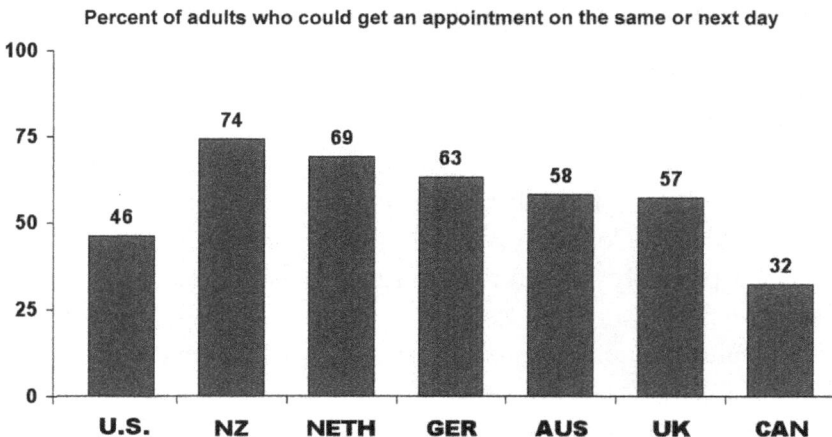

Source: The Commonwealth Fund Commission on a High Performance Health System. Why Not the Best? Results from the National Scorecard on U.S. Health System Performance. Vol. 97, July 17, 2008. Reprinted with permission.

- A 2008 report by the U.S. Centers for Disease Control and Prevention, based on a national survey of 362 hospital emergency rooms, found a 32 percent increase in ER visits between 1996 and 2006, with average waits to see a physician increasing from 38 minutes in 1997 to 56 minutes in 2006;[80] another recent study found that wait times in ERs for patients with acute heart attacks increased by an average of 11.2 percent a year from 1997 to 2004, with waits considerably longer for blacks, Hispanics, and women.[81]

- A 2007 survey by the American College of Emergency Physicians (ACEP) of almost 1,500 emergency physicians found that 13 percent had personally experienced a patient dying as a result of being "boarded" in a hallway in the emergency department while waiting for a hospital bed.[82] By late 2008, the ACEP was aware of at least 200 patients who had died on stretchers in hospital corridors while being "boarded" awaiting admission to the hospital.[83]

- Wait times are increasing for patients to see a primary care physician. In Massachusetts, for example, where we have discussed the "breakthrough reform" for universal coverage, the average wait time for a new patient to see an internist is now 50 days, with the longest wait being 100 days; the Massachusetts Medical Society has found that 42 percent of primary care physicians have stopped seeing new patients, up from 33 percent in 2004.[84]

- Uninsured adults in Los Angeles County face wait times up to a year or longer for gall bladder or hernia surgery; patients of the Southside Coalition of Community Health Centers in that county typically wait for 6 to 12 months for most specialty services.[85]

- The wait time debate usually comes down to comparisons with Canada. The Fraser Institute is an ultraconservative think tank in Vancouver, British Columbia, similar in ideology to the Dallas-based National Center for Policy Analysis (NCPA). It puts out misleading reports of excessive wait times in Canada. These reports are based on a definition of waiting times from when physicians *think* their patients will have to wait between referral from a family physician and specialty treatment, not their actual wait times.[86] But provincial analyses of waiting times show something different – that waits are not nearly as long as physicians think.[87]

As an example, the Fraser Institute reported that median wait times for surgery or specialty care was 17.8 weeks in 2003. Statistics Canada, however, the Canadian counterpart of the U.S. Census Bureau, reported that the median wait times across all provinces of Canada in 2003 were 4.0 weeks to see a specialist and 4.3 weeks for non-emergency surgery.[88] Major efforts have been made across Canada in recent years to reduce waiting times within their limited budget. In Ontario, for example, targets for waits from referral by the GP to a specialty consultant for radiation therapy of cancer have been set at 14 days, with targets for readiness to treat of 1, 7 and 14 days; more than one-half of cancer patients met these targets in August 2008, with two-thirds meeting the readiness to treat target.[89] In British Columbia, the mean visit time for radiation therapy for cancer patients is six days; virtually all patients are able to start chemotherapy within two weeks.[90]

- A 2006 population-based survey of more than 3,000 Canadians and 5,000 Americans found that only 3.5 percent of Canadians had unmet health care needs because of long waiting times, compared to 0.7 percent of Americans. But there is a flip side to that coin – 7 percent of Americans had unmet health care needs because of cost, compared to only 0.8 percent of Canadians.[91]

- Opponents of single-payer NHI in this country often point to the fact that Americans get hip replacement surgery done here much faster than Canadians do; this is humorous, since most Americans get that procedure done on our single-payer system – Medicare! This also should give us confidence that waiting times under single-payer NHI will not be excessive since we have more resources already invested in health care than is the case in Canada.

## 12. NHI will raise my taxes.

This myth spreads the fear that NHI will open the flood gates to spiraling health care costs, and that taxes will have to increase. For many, it further implies that we will have many low-income "freeloaders" and that we already pay high enough taxes today. But as we already saw in the last chapter, we have enough money in the system now to cover the costs of NHI by administrative simplification, reallocation of funds, and elimination of the wasteful bureaucracy of private insurers.[92]

Actually, on the "top end" of taxpayers, we are at relatively low levels of taxation by historical standards over the last 90 years, as shown by Figure 10.5.[93] At the "low end", we have regressive tax policies that hit low-income people much harder than higher-income Americans. According to the Congressional Budget Office, families with household incomes of $25,000 today spend 9 percent of their income on health care through taxes alone.[94] And as Princeton's Uwe Reinhardt reminds us, families with incomes between $20,000 and

FIGURE 10.5

# Changes in Top Tax Rate in the U.S. - 1918 to 2005

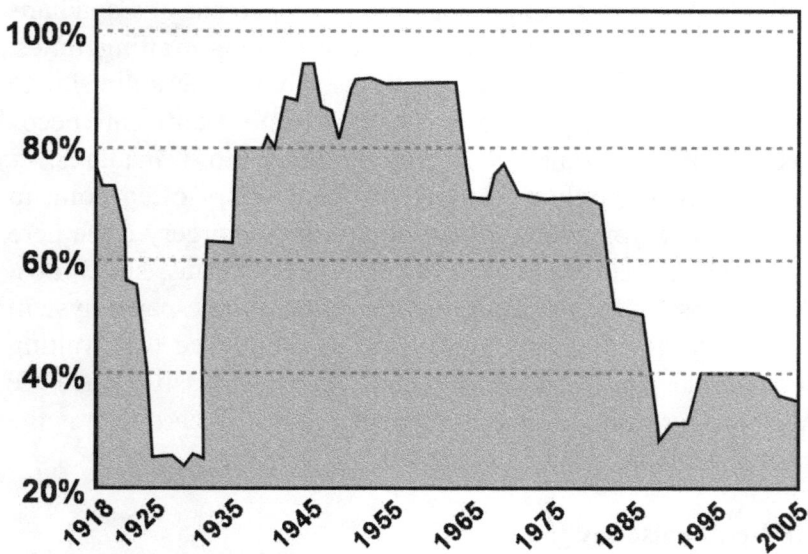

Source: Himmelstein DU. The National Health Program Slideshow Guide. Center for National Health Program Studies. Cambridge, MA, 2008. Reprinted with permission.

$60,000, about one-third of American households, were sailing into a perfect storm of health care costs even before what is likely to be a prolonged recession that started in 2008.[95]

As for value, NHI will give us universal coverage of necessary care for all Americans for the least amount of money, probably at levels less than what we are already paying. Many national surveys over the years have shown widespread and stable support for NHI. A 2005 survey by the Pew Research Center, for example, found that two-thirds of Americans support "government health insurance even if taxes increase," with high levels of support among many "conservative" respondents – "populist conservatives" (63 percent) and "conservative Democrats" (73 percent).[96]

The long-standing strong majority of popular support for NHI shows why those who favor the status quo work so hard to perpetuate myths and disinformation – they need to stoke confusion in the face of clarity about what is needed. And for us it suggests that the distance we must travel to overcome the myths is not as great as it sometimes appears.

As Paul Krugman points out:

"The bottom line is that the opponents of universal health care appear to have run out of honest arguments. All they have left is fantasies: horror fiction about health care in other countries, and fairy tales about health care here in America."[97]

We need to reframe the health care debate based on evidence, experience, traditional American values, and principles in keeping with the American Cancer Society's 4 As of coverage – adequate, affordable, available, and administratively simple. That is the subject of the next and last chapter, where we will also present an eight-point plan for improvement of cancer care within a reformed health care system.

# References:

1. www.brainyquote.com/quotes/quotes/a/abrahamlin110340.html.
2. Bradley B. *The New American Story*. New York. Random House.2007: p xiii.
3. Kennedy JF. Commencement Address. Yale University, June 11, 1962.

4.  Goodman JC, Herrick DM. Twenty Myths about Single-Payer Health Insurance: International Evidence on the Effects of National Health Insurance in Countries around the World. Dallas, TX. National Center for Policy Analysis, 2002: p 64.
5.  Public Citizen. Medicare Privatization: The Case Against Relying on the HMOs and Private Insurers to Offer Prescription Drug Coverage. Washington, D.C., 2002.
6.  General Accounting Office. Medicare + Choice: Payments Exceed Costs of Fee for Service Benefits, Adding Billions to Spending. GAO/HEHS-00-161. Washington, D. C.: Government Printing Office, 2000.
7.  Orszag PR. Testimony on the Medicare Advantage Program before the Committee on the Budget U.S. House of Representatives, June 28, 2007.
8.  GAO. Medicare Advantage: Increases spending relative to Medicare fee-for-service may not always reduce beneficiary out-of-pocket costs. Government Printing Office, February 2008.
9.  Gruber J. Tax policy for health insurance. National Bureau of Economic Research, December, 2004.
10. Fuhrmans V. Billing battle. Fights over health claims spawn a new arms race. *Wall Street Journal* , February 14, 2007: A1.
11. Fronstin P. Outlook on Consumerism in Health Care. Washington, D.C. Employee Benefit Research Institute (EBRI), 2008, p 9.
12. Market Watch. BlueCross BlueShield of Michigan answers attorney general. December 1, 2008.
13. Personal communication, Rob Stone, M.D., January 20, 2009.
14. Fuhrmans V. Long-term outlook for health insurers, Wall Street Journal, October 27, 2008, as cited in Kaiser Daily Health Policy Report, October 27, 2008.
15. Fuhrmans V. Health insurers sell off sharply on new Medicare payment rates. *Wall Street Journal*, February 24, 2009: B7.
16. Jannarone J. Health care gets a shock treatment. *Wall Street Journal*, February, 27, 2009: C 10.
17. Becker C. One question: credit or debt? As health savings accounts gain in popularity, insurers and the financial services industry want to bank the cash. *Mod Healthcare* 36: 6-16, 2006.
18. AHIP. About AHIP. Web site accessed September 16, 2007.
19. Terhune C. Thin cushion. Fast-growing health plan has a catch, $1,000 a year cap. *Wall Street Journal* , May 14, 2003: A1.
20. Commonwealth Fund. Many with insurance lack choice. New York. Issue Brief, 2005.
21. Associated Press. Study: Health insurers are near monopolies. April 18, 2006.
22. Robinson JC. Consolidation and the transformation of competition in health insurance. *Health Affairs (Millwood)* 23 (6): 11-24, 2004.
23. The Commonwealth Fund Commission on a High Performance Health System. Why Not the Best? Results from the National Scorecard on U.S. Health System Performance. Vol. 97, July 17, 2008.
24. Associated Press. U.S. ranks just 42nd in life expectancy. Lack of insurance, obesity, social disparities to blame, experts say. August 11, 2007.

25. Guyatt GH, Devereaux PJ, Lexchin J, et al. A systematic review of studies comparing health outcomes in Canada and the United States. *Open Medicine* 1 (1), 2007.
26. Gorey KM, et al. An international comparison of cancer survival: Toronto, Ontario and Detroit, Michigan metropolitan areas. *Am J Public Health* 87: 1156-63, 1997.
27. Banks J, Marmot M, Oldfield Z, et al. Disease and disadvantage in the United States and England. *JAMA* 295: 2037-45, 2006.
28. Starfield B, Shi L. The medical home, access to care, and insurance: a review of evidence. *Pediatrics* 113: 1493-98, 2004.
29. Starfield B. *Primary Care: Concept, Evaluation and Policy.* Oxford University Press. New York, 1992.
30. Roetzheim RG, Pal N, Gonzalez EC, et al. The effects of physician supply on the early detection of colorectal cancer. *J Fam Pract* 48 (11): 850-8, 1999.
31. Geyman JP. *The Corrosion of Medicine: Can the Profession Reclaim its Moral Legacy?* Monroe, ME. Common Courage Press, 2008, p37.
32. Cherlin, EJ, Carlson, MA, Herrin, J, Schulman-Green, D, Barry, CL et al. Interdisciplinary staffing patterns: Do for-profit and nonprofit hospices differ? Journal of Palliative Medicine 13 (4): 389-94, 2010.
33. Wennberg JB, Fisher ES, Skinner JS. Geography and the debate over Medicare reform. *Health Affairs Web Exclusive* W-103, February 13, 2002.
34. Fisher ES, Wennberg DE, Stukel TA, et al. The implications of regional variations in Medicare spending. Part 2: Health outcomes and satisfaction with care. *Ann Intern Med* 138 ($): 288-98, 2003.
35. Starfield B. Access, primary care, and the medical home; rights of passage. *Medical Care* 46 (10): 1016, 2008.
36. Evans RG. Separate and unequal: self-segregation in health insurance. *Medical Care* 46 (10): 1014, 2008.
37. Woolhandler S, Day B, Himmelstein DU. State health reform flatlines. *Intl J Health Services* 38 (3): 585-92, 2008.
38. Nardin R, Himmelstein DU, Woolhandler S. Press Release. Massachusett's Plan: A failed model for health care reform. Washington, DC. February, 18, 2009.
39. Sack K. With health care for nearly all, Massachusetts now faces costs. *New York Times,* March 16, 2009:A1.
40. U.S. Department of Health and Human Services. Office of the National Coordinator for Health Information Technology. May 23, 2005. http://www.hhs.gov/healthit/valueHIT.html, accessed April 27, 2006.
41. GAO (U.S. Government Accountability Office). Statement of David A Powner. Testimony Before the Subcommittee on Federal Workforce and Agency Organization, Committee on Government Reform, House of Representatives Health Information Technology. HHS is Continuing Efforts to Define Its National Strategy, September 1, 2006.
42. GAO. Report to Congressional Committee on Domestic and Offshore Outsourcing of Personal Information in Medicare, Medicaid, and TRICARE, September, 2006.

43. Wang SJ, Middleton B, Prosser LA, et al. A cost-benefit analysis of electronic medical records in primary care. *Am J Med* 114 (5): 397-403, 2003.
44. Sidorov J. It ain't necessarily so: The electronic health record and the unlikely prospect of reducing health care costs. *Health Aff (Millwood)* 25 (4): 1179-85, 2006.
45. Hoffman C, Rice D, Sung, HY. Persons with chronic conditions: Their prevalence and costs. *JAMA* 276 (18): 1473-79, 1996.
46. Holtz-Eakin P. CBO Director. Testimony to Congress. October 13, 2004.
47. Mattke S, Seid M, Ma S. Evidence for the effect of disease management: Is $1 billion a year a good investment? *Am J Manag Care* 13: 670-76, 2007.
48. American Diabetes Association. High-risk pools. Health Insurance Resource Manual. Alexandria, VA, 2006.
49. Families USA. AHPs: Bad medicine for small employers. Washington, D. C.: December, 2005.
50. Baumgardner J, Hagen S. Increasing Small Firm Health Insurance Coverage Through Association Health Plans and Health Marts. Washington, D. C.: Congressional Budget Office, January, 2000.
51. Geyman JP. *Do Not Resuscitate: Why The Health Insurance Industry Is Dying, and How We Must Replace It.* Monroe, ME. Common Courage Press, 2008, pp 137-44.
52. Himmelstein DU. Presentation at the Annual Meeting of Physicians for a National Health Program, San Diego, CA, October 25, 2008.
53. Milliman Medical Index, 2008. Accessed on November 10, 2008 at http://www.milliman.com/expertise/healthcare/products-tools/mmi/pdfs/milliman-medical-indes-2008.pdf.
54. Evans RG. Separate and unequal: self-segregation in health insurance. *Medical Care* 46 (10): 1014, 2008.
55. Carrasquillo O, Himmelstein DU, Woolhandler S, et al. A reappraisal off private employers' role in providing health insurance. *N Engl J Med* 340 (2): 109-14, 1999.
56. Editorial. Health care by loopholes. *AARP Bulletin* 48 (3): 3, 2007.
57. Gross D. National health care? We're halfway there. *New York Times*, December 3, 2006.
58. Woolhandler S. Interview. Unhealthy solutions: Private insurance, high cost and the denial of care. *Multinational Monitor,* September/October, 2008.
59. Krugman P. Bailouts for bunglers. *New York Times*, February 2, 2009: A 19.
60. Himmelstein DU. The National Health Program Slide-Show Guide. Center for National Health Program Studies. Cambridge, MA, 2000.
61. Krugman P. The world of U.S. health care economics is downright scary. *Seattle Post-Intelligencer*, September 26, 2006: B1.
62. Kahn JG, Kronick R, Kryer M, et al. The cost of health insurance administration in California: estimates for insurers, physicians, and hospitals. *Health Aff (Millwood)* 24 (6): 1629, 2005.
63. Kagel R. Blue crossroads: Insurance in the 21st Century. *American Medical News*, September 20, 2004.

64. Survey reveals that doctors feel pressured by health insurers to alter the way they treat patients. The Medical Society of the State of New York, September 2, 2008.
65. Morra, D, Nicholson, S, Levinson, W, Gans, DN, Hammons, T et al. U.S. physician practices versus Canadians: Spending nearly four times as much money interacting with payers. *Health Affairs* 30 (8): 1443-9, 2011.
66. Angell M. *The Truth About the Drug Companies: How They Deceive Us and What We Can Do About It.* New York. Random House. 2004, pp 234-5.
67. Blue Cross and Blue Shield. Technology Evaluation Committee Reports, No. 1-28, 1999.
68. Ibid #60, 2008, based on OECD figures for 2006.
69. Light DW, Lexchin J. Foreign free riders and the high price of U.S. medicines. *BMJ* 331: 958-60, 2005.
70. GAO. NIH-Private Sector Partnership in the Development of Taxol. Washington, D. C. General Accounting Office, 2003. Available at www.gao.gov/cgi-bin/getrpt?GAO-03-829.
71. Nyman JA. *The Theory of Demand for Health Insurance.* Stanford, CA. Stanford University Press, 2003.
72. Nyman JA. Is "moral hazard" inefficient? The policy implications of a new theory. *Health Aff (Millwood)* 23 (5): 194-99, 2004.
73. Ibid #22.
74. Goldman DP, Joyce GF, Zheng Y. Prescription drug cost-sharing: associations with medication and medical utilization and spending and health. *JAMA* 298 (11): 61-88, 2007.
75. Artiga S, O'Malley M. Increasing premiums and cost-sharing in Medicaid and SCHIP: Recent state experiences. Issue Paper. Kaiser Commission on Medicaid and the Uninsured. Kaiser Family Foundation, May 2005, p2.
76. Armstrong P, Armstrong H, Fegan C. *Universal Health Care: What the United States Can Learn from the Canadian Experience.* New York. The New Press, 1998, p 131.
77. Greg L, Stoddard GL, et al. Why Not User Charges? The Real Issues, a discussion paper prepared for the (Ontario) Premier's Council on Health, Well-being and Social Justice, September, 1993, pp 5-6.
78. Ibid # 4, p 95.
79. Ibid # 22.
80. Pitts S. CDC: Average ER wait time approaches one hour. Atlanta, GA, August 6, 2008.
81. Wilper A, Woolhandler S, Lasser KE, et al. Waits to see an emergency department physician: U.S. trends and predictors, 1997 – 2004, *Health Aff (Millwood)* 27 (2): W 84-W95, 2008.
82. Johnson CK. 'Halfway medicine' seen as a way to unclutter ERs. *Houston Chronicle/AP* , October, 26, 2008.
83. Abelson R. Uninsured put stress on hospitals. *New York Times*, December 9, 2008: B1.
84. Kowalezyk L. Across Mass: wait to see doctors grows. *Boston Globe,* September, 22, 2008.

85. Engel M. Uninsured adults face yearlong delays for some surgeries. *Los Angeles Times*, July 25, 2007.

86. Esmail N, Walker M. Waiting your turn: hospital waiting lists in Canada (14th edition, 2004. Available at http://www.fraserinstitute.ca/shared/readmore.asp?sNav=pb&id=705.

87. DeCoster C, et al. Waiting Times for Surgery: 1997/98 and 1998/99 Update: Manitoba Centre for Health Policy and Evaluation. Available at http://www.umanitoba.ca/centres/mchp/reports/pdfs/waits2.pdf.

88. Canadian Health Services Research Foundation Newsletter. Vol. 1 No. 4, available at www.chsrf.ca.

89. Radiation treatment wait times, August, 2008, for Ontario. Available at http://www.cancercare.on.ca/english/home/ocs/wait-times/radiationwt/ (accessed on November 19, 2008).

90. Wait times for cancer services. Ministry of Health, Government of British Columbia. Accessed March 10, 2009 at http://www.healthservices.gov.bc.ca/wait-list/cancer.html.

91. Lasser KE, Himmelstein DU, Woolhandler S. Access to care, health status, and health disparities in the United States and Canada: Results of a cross-national population-based survey. *Am J Public Health* 46 (7): 1-8, 2006.

92. Woolhandler S. Interview. Unhealthy solutions: Private insurance, high cost and the denial of care. *Multinational Monitor,* September/October, 2008, p 38.

93. Ibid # 60, 2008.

94. Harrison, JA. Paying more, getting less. *Dollars & Sense*. May/June 2008.

95. Reinhardt UE. The health care challenge: sailing into a perfect storm. *New York Times*, November 7, 2008.

96. Pew Research Center. Beyond Red vs, Blue. Survey Report, May 10, 2005.

97. Krugman P. The waiting game. *New York Times*, Jul y 16, 2007: A17.

CHAPTER 11

# A Way to Win:
# An Eight-Point Plan Based on
# National Health Insurance

"There is no reason why, in a society which has reached the general level of wealth ours has, [the certainty of a given minimum of sustenance] should not be guaranteed to all without endangering general freedom; that is: some level of food, shelter and clothing, sufficient to preserve health. Nor is there any reason why the state should not help to organize a comprehensive system of social insurance in providing for those common hazards of life against which few can make adequate provision."[1]

—Dr. Friedrich A. Hayek, 1962
Professor of Social and Moral Sciences, University of Chicago
(1950-1962) Neuroscientist, leading conservative economist of
his time, author of the classic *The Road to Serfdom*, and Nobel
laureate in Economics in 1974

"Knowing is not enough; we must apply. Willing is not enough; we must do."

—Johann Wolfgang von Goethe (1749-1832)
Leading man of letters, scientist, humanist and philosopher

There is no way that private insurance can be relied upon to protect us from cancer, what is becoming the leading cause of death in this country, as it already is for Americans under 85. The way we pay for cancer care is killing us, both financially and literally. We have a two (or more)-tiered system within which lower-income people and those of ethnic minorities get second or third-rate care while the best care is the domain of the rich. Many examples in earlier chapters bear witness to the pain and suffering that devastates so many American families with cancer.

Time is running out for the Baby Boomer generation, now on a collision course with their rising cancer risk and a system that increasingly excludes them from adequate care. The persistent question is this: Can we rebuild our failing health care system fast enough to avoid sacrificing many in this generation?

In the previous chapter we looked at many of the myths that have stood in the way of serious reform for many years. We are still in a policy vacuum concerning health care reform, with a contentious battle continuing to play out across the political spectrum as the 2011-12 election cycle heats up.

Though he was a leading light for conservatives in the last century, Dr. Hayek had serious concerns about the damage that can be wrought by unrestrained markets. We can expect that he would be appalled at how far deregulated health care markets have gone in our time, as documented in the preceding chapters for such a major problem as cancer care. And as Goethe points out, it's time to act.

This chapter has four goals: (1) to reframe the health care debate based on principles and values; (2) to sketch out an eight-step plan to improve cancer care within overall health care reform; (3) to summarize a paradigm shift that will be needed in U.S. health care if all cancer patients are to have affordable access to effective care in the future; and (4) to briefly consider the changing political landscape that will bear on whether and how health care reform is likely to unfold.

## Reframing the Health Care Debate

Market advocates and conservative legislators and policy makers have for years framed the health care debate to their advantage, proclaiming the presumed efficiencies of private markets to solve our problems, together with other myths as described in the previous chapter. They raise the specter of "government control", "socialized medicine" and runaway costs if single-payer public financing is enacted.

As we saw in Chapter 9 (Table 9.4), a publicly-financed single-payer system (NHI) is an excellent fit with traditional American values, as opposed to private health insurance, which is not. It's about fairness, efficiency, accountability for access and quality, fiscal responsibility, and eliminating waste and profiteering on the backs of vulnerable sick people, our fellow citizens. It's about sharing the risks of disease and injury across our whole population, putting us all together in the same boat, in one tier of care.

There is a wide political divide separating advocates of the unfettered medical marketplace in a multi-payer financing system from proponents of a public-financing system with NHI and a private delivery system. Both sides espouse many of the same values, such as freedom, individual responsibility, and the American spirit of entrepreneurialism. But their paths diverge sharply when it comes to their interpretations of these values. Free market advocates, for example, prefer government to have a minimal custodial role, and specifically reject the United Nations' Universal Declaration of Human Rights, which states: "Everyone has the right to a standard of living adequate for the health and well-being of himself and his family, including food, clothing, housing and medical care and necessary social services."[2]

In their 2007 Rockridge Institute Report, *The Logic of the Health Care Debate*, University of California linguist George Lakoff and his colleagues analyzed and compared three types of political thought – conservative, progressive and neoliberal. They made the case that single-payer NHI is an economically and morally superior approach to financing health care, and suggested these progressive requirements for a health care system:[3]

"• Everyone should have access to comprehensive, quality health care (follows from empathy).
• No one should be denied care for the sake of private profit (follows from empathy and protection).
• You can choose your own doctor (follows from empathy).
• Promotion of health and well-being, focusing on preventive care (follows from individual responsibility).
• Costs should be progressive, that is, readily affordable to everyone, with higher costs borne by those better able to pay (follows from empathy).
• Access should be extremely easy, with no specific roadblocks (follows from responsibility).
• Administration should be simple and cheap (follows from empathy and responsibility).

- Interactions should be minimally bureaucratic and maximally human (follows from empathy and responsibility).
- Payments should be adequate for doctors, nurses, and other health care workers. Conditions of their employment should be reasonable (follows from empathy)."

Single-payer NHI meets all of these requirements, as enabled by other reform steps to be discussed below. Multi-payer financing will never get us there, no matter how we try to tweak that system.

Boiled down to its essence, the health care debate is about the private interest versus the public interest, and an individual versus a societal perspective. Does one side trump the other? And, if not, where is the balance between these two poles? Dr. Don McCanne, who practiced many years in Orange County, California, before serving two years as President of Physicians for a National Health Program (PNHP), has this to say on this crucial matter:

"Freedom, entrepreneurialism, and individual responsibility are values that are not the exclusive domain of the opponents of single-payer, for we all share them. The disagreement is in how we value public policies that make these concepts work for all of us. We need freedom – freedom to choose our health care professionals – a freedom that the insurers have taken away from us. We need entrepreneurialism to provide us with better technology – but technology that meets the test of value. We need to exercise our individual responsibility to take care of ourselves – but along with our responsibility to support public policies that will enhance the health of all of us."[4]

For me, reframing our goals for health care reform can be quite simple:

"Restore the promise of opportunity and security by promoting better health of our people, communities and country through enlightened health policies of fiscal prudence and fairness to all."[5]

# An Eight-Step Approach
# Toward One-Tier Cancer Care

These eight steps will go a long way toward making the American Cancer Society's goal of 4 As a reality. These steps are just sketched out here with the intent to suggest the dimensions of the challenges facing real health care reform. The issues are complex, but each of these steps is integral to a coherent strategy to make affordable and effective cancer care available to all cancer patients in this country.

**1. Enact universal coverage through National Health Insurance.**
This has to be the most important and absolutely essential first step upon which to build other needed improvements in cancer care. Without NHI, unaccountable private insurers will continue to cherry pick the market, divide the risk pool, increase costs of care for everyone, and saddle beleaguered public programs with unsustainable costs of financing care for sicker people. We cannot continue to expose our fellow citizens who are unfortunate enough to get cancer, now or in the future, to the perils of the market and the catastrophic costs of their care. Nor can we in good conscience set up two or three tiers of care, based on ability to pay, which leave most cancer patients without adequate care.

Although we pay much more for health care than any other country in the world, we get little return for it as a society. A 2008 report, *Measure of America*, puts some new numbers on where we now stand in the world. Funded by Oxfam America, the Conrad Hilton Foundation and the Rockefeller Foundation, the American Human Development Report applies rankings of health, education, and income to the U.S., including calculations for our overall human development index (HDI). This index was developed by Nobel laureate economist Amartya Sen in 1990, who had this to say at the time: "Human development is concerned with what I take to be the basic development idea: namely, advancing the richness of human life, rather than the richness of the economy in which human beings live, which is only a part of it." Here are some of the findings of this 2008 report:[6]

- Despite spending more than $5 billion a day on health care and having the second-highest per capita income in the world, the U.S. ranks 42nd in terms of life expectancy.
- Although we are still the world's leading economy, we have dropped from 2nd in human development in 1990 to 12th place today.
- This country has a higher percentage of children living in poverty than any of the world's richest countries.
- About 40 million Americans lack the literacy skills to perform simple everyday tasks, such as understanding newspaper articles
- Income inequality is stark; the richest 20 percent of Americans have an average annual income of $168,170, almost 15 times that of the lowest 20 percent ($11,352).

Kristen Lewis of the American Human Development Project draws this overall conclusion: "For Americans to live longer, healthier lives as well as to remain solvent when serious illness strikes, it is obvious from this report that progress depends in large part on a comprehensive resolution of the problem of health insurance."[7]

As we saw in the last chapter, taxpayers are already financing two-thirds of all health care spending in this country, much more than most people realize.[8,9] As private insurers face declining private markets, accelerated in our economic downturn, they are turning to the taxpayer for still more help. They are already subsidized by hundreds of billions of dollars a year through tax exemptions and government overpayments. Now, in their death spiral as an industry, AHIP has called for mandated health insurance, even to the point of guaranteed issue.[10] Guaranteed issue really means that the industry wants still more government subsidies, requiring more people to buy its coverage with more taxpayer money. Nowhere in the equation is industry willing to accept controls over its pricing and coverage policies, or acknowledge its many inefficiencies and enormous burden of administrative and overhead costs. Public financing, provided on a not-for-profit basis without the high costs of product design, medical underwriting and marketing that are carried out by private insurers, remains much more efficient in offering value of coverage that we can depend on.

NHI is not the answer to all of our problems, but it is an essential first step. For cancer as well as other health care, it can provide a structure for other needed improvements to take place (Table 11.1). Dr. Laura Boylan, neurologist at the New York University School of Medicine, sees single-payer Medicare for All as the obvious way to deal with our crisis in health care:

---

### TABLE 11.1

## AN EIGHT-POINT PLAN
## FOR ONE-TIER CANCER CARE

1. Enact single-payer national health insurance, Medicare-for-All
2. Establish a national science-based Clinical Effectiveness Program
3. Broaden focus and increase public funding for cancer research
4. Expand the use of evidence-based practice guidelines
5. Revise reimbursement policies to rebuild primary care and minimize perverse incentives among providers
6. Strengthen cancer workforce, especially in primary care and geriatric oncology
7. Address ethical issues in cancer care and research
8. Empower regulators to provide oversight and accountability of best products and practices

---

"In the face of economic collapse and soaring unemployment, with a third of Americans foregoing medical care due to cost, 'Job No. 1' is getting value for our health care dollar, not preserving employer-based health insurance. The repetition of failed experiments is not pragmatic, it is part tragedy and part farce. Electronic medical records, chronic disease management and more emphasis on prevention are all important for many reasons but we must admit that short- and long-term implications are unknown. Some of these measures may actually increase costs. Medicare is not perfect, but it is demonstrably more cost-effective than private insurance and beloved by most Americans. It is 'shovel ready.' Single-payer supporters say: everybody in, nobody out."[11]

**2. Establish a national science-based Clinical Effectiveness Program to better focus our resources.**

Peter Orszag, former White House budget director, has estimated that we could save as much as $700 billion a year by not paying for services that lack good clinical outcomes.[12] Such a colossal savings would change the landscape of how we fight not only cancer but other diseases as well.

As noted in Chapters 2 and 3, this has been a difficult challenge for our country to deal with, and we have failed over many years to limit developing technologies on the basis of clinical effectiveness or cost-benefit. As a nation beholden to the glamour of new technology, we allow industry and markets to largely control what is adopted into clinical practice, often with limited supporting scientific evidence. Manufacturers, hospitals and physicians who stand to benefit financially from early adoption, lobbyists and other intermediaries between industry and policy makers, all push for rapid adoption of new products. Payers, whether Medicare or private insurers, are pressured by market forces to make coverage and reimbursement decisions before much evidence is available. Medicare, as the main trendsetter for these decisions, still has its hands tied by law (since 1965 it has been prevented from using cost-effectiveness criteria in its coverage policies). The FDA as well is hobbled by industry (which supports much of its budget through user fees) and by political interference from legislators responding to lobbyists.

The challenges are real, as illustrated by the current boom in advanced medical imaging, including CT, MRI and PET scanning. A recent report by the Medicare Payment Advisory Commission (MedPAC) found that the volume in imaging procedures per Medicare beneficiary has been exceeding the growth of all other services physicians provide.[13] There are now more than 7,000 sites in the country offering MRI, each unit costing some $2 million. With each new MRI unit, imaging procedures go up by more than 2,200 per year at a cost of $685,000 in additional spending.[14] There is very little evidence that this boom adds much value to care, and many experts are quite sure that much of this imaging is unnecessary and even harmful when we take into account the cumulative risks of radiation exposure.[15] Not surprisingly, this is another area of widespread conflicts of interest. Manufacturers welcome this boom, while hospitals and outpatient imaging centers find imaging to be a lucrative revenue center. Many physicians have an ownership stake in these centers, and profit through self-referral. We still have no effective ways to rein in overuse or to contain costs in this area.

So far, we have very limited ways of dealing with these problems. Medicare, as a single-payer system for 43 million Americans, has been developing a "coverage with evidence development" (CED) system to make some of its coverage decisions based on clinical evidence, but this is still quite limited.[16] And Peter Orszag, former White House budget director, recognizes the potential impact of reimbursement policy in reining in inappropriate services, with this observation:

"The Medicare program has not taken costs into account in determining what services are covered and has made only limited use of data on comparative effectiveness in its payment policies; but if statutory changes permitted it, Medicare could use information about comparative effectiveness to promote higher-value care. For example, Medicare could tie its payments to providers to the cost of the most effective or most efficient treatment. If that payment was less than the cost of providing a more expensive service, then doctors and hospitals would probably elect not to provide it – so the change in Medicare's payment policy would have the same practical effect as a coverage decision."[17]

We are an outlier in the world among advanced countries in not having an effective mechanism to make coverage and reimbursement policies informed by science and cost-effectiveness, but we can look to other countries for many examples of how to do it. The United Kingdom's National Institute for Health and Clinical Excellence (NICE) is a leading example,[18] as is Canada's Common Drug Review.[19]

The Affordable Care Act of 2010 did create a non-profit Patient-Centered Outcomes Research Institute to be charged with examining the relative outcomes, clinical effectiveness and appropriateness of different medical treatments. But it will not have the power to mandate or even endorse coverage or reimbursement rules for any particular treatment. So the priority for establishing remains urgent. Whatever the name of such a new national institution that is established to fulfill this role, we already know that it has to have an adequate budget and staff, scientific expertise, authority and independence from political interference, and a societal perspective.

## 3. Broaden Focus and Increase Public Funding for Cancer Research.

Although the National Cancer Institute (NCI) is a world-class leader in cancer research, its activities are limited by funding and by the kinds of research projects brought to it by applicants. Industry supports more than twice the amount of biomedical research financed by the National Institutes of Health (57 percent vs. 28 percent in 2003).[20] While some would tout this as a success, we pay a high price for limiting public funding as severely as we do. The current world of cancer research is rife with conflicts of interest throughout the research process, ranging from the kinds of questions that are investigated to methods and protocols of study, and to reporting or non-reporting of end results. The interests of industry, of course, are driven by the potential of future profits and protection of their patents for new products. As a result, some important clinical questions that are not likely to be profitable are not studied, while others of limited scientific value are studied for their market potential.

These are some of the areas that have not as yet received enough attention, and each would benefit from increased funding:

- cancer prevention
- cancer screening
- watchful waiting (e.g. for prostate cancer)
- drug vs. drug studies
- cancer in the elderly

Shifting to a much larger share of public financing for cancer research could help to steer research toward important clinical questions and provide increased oversight of research integrity, rigor and accountability. Dean Baker, Ph.D., Co-Director at the Washington, D.C.-based Center for Economic and Policy Research, has recently proposed a novel idea – public financing of clinical drug trials by contracting with private sector companies to conduct the trials. The cost of the trials would be about $20 billion dollars, according to figures from 2007. Under his proposal, these costs would be more than recovered by savings brought about by CMS negotiating discounts of prescription drugs under Part D of the Medicare program. This process would be similar to what the Veterans Administration already does. Benefits of this proposal include:[21]

- projected savings of some $50 billion over a 10-year period for the costs of trials
- bringing more rigor to the research process
- reducing much of the wasted resources now being expended on the development of copy-cat drugs of little clinical value,
- elimination of many of the conflicts-of-interest now inherent in drug research
- substantial efficiency gains for society.

Baker suggests that any of several federal agencies could contract out research projects, whether the NIH, FDA, CMS, or another agency such as a new Comparative Effectiveness Institute mentioned above.

Randomized clinical trials, while the gold standard for many basic research studies, are not appropriate for many important and practical questions. Many advocates in the research and policy communities are now recommending that we develop mechanisms to fund and conduct many more pragmatic trials, while retaining scientific rigor appropriate to the questions being studied.

Dr. David Kessler, former FDA Commissioner, and others have proposed that the process of cancer clinical trials could be accelerated by using "progression-free survival" (PFS) as a surrogate end point. PFS measures the progression of cancer receiving experimental treatment. Advocates believe that use of this measure instead of death as an endpoint could speed up cancer clinical trials, as it already has done in AIDS research.[22] Many oncologists, however, find this endpoint too "soft" and dependent on the timing of testing. Dr. Steven Goodman, oncologist and biostatistician at Johns Hopkins School of Medicine, further recommends that pragmatic trials should be as simple as possible, measuring such outcomes as hospitalizations and deaths, not trying to answer why these outcomes occurred.[23] Ideally, most if not all cancer patients should be in some kind of trial, with transparency of results being monitored through the widespread use of cancer registries.

Enrollment of cancer patients in clinical trials has been limited for many years by difficulties that patients and their physicians have in finding applicable trials. Many pervasive myths have surrounded the subject of clinical trials. One important myth held by many people is that placebos may be used in their treatment. But Dr. Robert Comis, who heads Drexel University's Clinical Trials Research Center, reassures us that: "If there is a standard of care for a particular type of cancer, we'd never use a placebo in lieu of that standard of care, though a placebo might be used in addition to standard-of-care treatment."[24]

A non-profit Coalition of Cancer Cooperative Groups has developed TrialCheck as a tool that can be used to search for trials by type of cancer and zip code. It includes all available trials by the National Cancer Institute, other government agencies, the Cancer Cooperative Group, and the drug/biotech industries. It is further described in Appendix 2.[25]

## 4. Expand the use of evidence-based clinical practice guidelines.

As the volume of medical information expands at an ever increasing pace, beyond what most clinicians can keep up with, clinical practice guidelines (CPGs) have played a growing role in encouraging the best and latest clinical practice across all fields of medicine. CPGs have proliferated since the 1990s, promulgated by specialty organizations, governmental agencies, and other groups.

The quality of CPGs still varies considerably, depending on the scientific rigor whereby they are developed, the quality of the scientific evidence brought to bear, and the objectivity of the group involved. At their best, they provide practicing physicians with unbiased recommendations informed by the latest scientific evidence as assessed by researchers and expert clinicians. But we still need to guard against accepting CPGs that are tainted by conflicts-of-interest with industry and market interests among those developing the guidelines. Of 100 authors of 44 CPGs endorsed by North American and European societies on common adult diseases between 1991 and 1999, for example, 59 percent of the authors had personal financial relationships (mostly undisclosed) with drug companies whose drugs were being considered in guidelines they authored.[26] Unfortunately, the conflict-of-interest problem is still with us more than a decade later. A 2011 study found that 81 percent of the leaders of groups writing 17 guidelines for the American Heart Association and the American College of Cardiology had personal financial interests in companies affected by their guidelines. [27]

As a cancer patient seeking care anywhere in the country, you should rightfully expect to receive the latest effective care. But how does your physician know what that is? Fortunately, there are now many highly respected sources of useful CPGs that can guide your physicians toward best current practice. CPGs, especially with a single-payer system utilizing the recommendations of a Comparative Effectiveness Institute (or a similar independent, non-partisan and not-for-profit agency), can help to reduce the present geographic variations in the quality of care and cut the costs of inappropriate and unnecessary services. Reimbursement for services can be tied to best practices, with denial of payment for medical mistakes (as CMS already does) and outlier services that fall short of currently recommended best practice.

The National Comprehensive Cancer Network (NCCN) is a not-for-profit alliance of 21 of the world's leading cancer centers. It has developed a compendium of clinical practice guidelines based on independent peer-reviewed evaluation of available scientific evidence. These guidelines have been adopted by some insurers (e.g., UnitedHealthcare) as well as CMS for Medicare as a guide for decisions concerning the coverage of cancer drugs and biologics.[28] But this is only a start to meet the need. Concerning the growing numbers of Baby Boomers being diagnosed with and living longer with cancer, a group of researchers recently had this to say about CPGs:

> "There is an urgent need for clear, evidence-based guidelines to assist physicians, oncologists and others who provide short- and long-term care management to older adults with cancer. Only with more immediate research will proper prevention efforts, screening, treatment approaches, post-treatment survivorship and end of life care be put in place to serve this rapidly growing population."[29]

## 5. Revise reimbursement policies to rebuild primary care and minimize perverse incentives among providers.

As we have seen in earlier chapters, the present reimbursement system gives perverse financial incentives to providers throughout our market-based system to offer inappropriate, unnecessary, and even harmful services that add to providers' bottom lines. This compromises the quality of care, leads to unrestrained escalation of health care costs, growing maldistribution of physicians by specialty, and a continued decline in primary care, the front line of cancer care.

It doesn't have to be this way. The way we reimburse health care services is largely a matter of historical artifact, dating back to the mid-1960s. As we recall from Chapter 8, a corporate compromise was struck at that time between the government, employers, physicians and hospitals whereby generous and permissive reimbursement arrangements would be allowed through Blue Cross as the lead fiscal intermediary for Medicare. These arrangements were based on "reasonable and customary" charges, which varied considerably from one part of the country to another, and strongly favored procedures over more time-intensive cognitive services typical in such fields as primary care, geriatrics, and psychiatry.[30]

A more recent example illustrates how hidden details of reimbursement policies drive up the costs of care and encourage inappropriate care. Beyond fees for their time and skills, Medicare reimburses physicians for their practice overhead expenses in providing specific services, such as rent, staff salaries, and the cost of high-tech equipment. In the case of CT scanning, for example, these expenses include some of the costs of purchase or leasing of the CT scanner. So the increased use of CT scanning becomes a lucrative revenue center. Not surprisingly, physicians order an estimated $40 billion worth of unnecessary imaging services each year.[31]

Reimbursement reform, as enabled by single-payer NHI and an agency like a Comparative Effectiveness Institute, can be a powerful tool to rein in the costs of care while improving its quality. Elements of this reform should include:

- Increased reimbursement for "medical homes" in primary care (see Glossary), as well as for time-intensive cognitive services in such specialties as geriatrics and psychiatry
- Decreased reimbursement for procedural services, in keeping with their value
- Decreased use of fee-for-service, with increased salaried practice, especially in groups

- Elimination of "balanced billing" (charges by physicians to patients beyond what payers pay)
- Non-payment for medically inappropriate or unnecessary services
- Ban on self-referral to facilities owned by physicians (e.g. specialty hospitals, imaging centers)
- Transition over time to a not-for-profit system

Dr. Arnold Relman, former editor of *The New England Journal of Medicine* and author of *A Second Opinion: Rescuing America's Health Care,* wisely observes:

"So long as private, for-profit companies handle the insurance, and so long as physicians and hospitals are driven by income-maximizing incentives that reward inefficiency and overutilization of resources, rising costs will continue to be at the center of our health care problem."[32]

**6. Strengthen the cancer workforce, especially in primary care and geriatric oncology.**

The cancer care workforce is shrinking, especially in primary care and geriatrics. The American College of Physicians has warned that "primary care, the backbone of the nation's health care system, is at grave risk of collapse."[33] Moreover, the Institute of Medicine has documented an acute shortage of geriatricians as the Baby Boomer generation nears retirement.[34]

The nation's supply of oncologists is also far short of projected future needs. In 2007 the *Journal of Oncology Practice* reported a study commissioned by the American Society of Clinical Oncology (ASCO) on the supply of and demand for oncology services in 2020. The study concluded that demand for oncology services will increase by 48 percent by 2020, mostly as a result of an 81 percent increase in cancer survivorship and a 48 percent increase in cancer incidence due to aging of the population. Although the number of oncologists is expected to grow by 14 percent by then, a shortfall of 2,550 to 4,080 oncologists is projected for 2020, about one-fourth to one-third of the 2005 supply of oncologists.[35] So critical shortages are occurring in primary care, geriatrics and oncology just when a larger workforce is becoming a more pressing need to deal with the growing prevalence of cancer.

No more than 30 percent of U.S. physicians are in primary care, and their numbers are continuing to decline as graduating medical students opt for higher-paying specialties with more controllable life styles.[36] Many patients are having a hard time finding a primary care physician. In Massachusetts, for example, where strong efforts have been made to expand access to care, only 51 percent of internists are accepting new patients and 95 percent of general physicians on the staffs of Boston's top three teaching hospitals have closed their practices to new patients.[37]

Without an adequate primary care base, the system becomes increasingly fragmented, inefficient, and overspecialized. Costs become uncontrollable. The quality of care drops. Disparities in health increase. Underserved populations are especially at risk, as the recruitment of primary care physicians to community health centers becomes even more difficult.[38]

While these system wide changes affect everyone, the lack of primary care is especially dangerous for cancer survivors. Those who are followed only by cancer specialists without also receiving care from primary care physicians have lower quality of care.[39]

Shoring up the cancer workforce will require a concerted and coordinated national strategy implemented over a long-term basis. Elements of this strategy, among others, should include reimbursement reform, building the "medical home" concept in primary care, loan forgiveness programs for medical students opting for primary care (their debts on graduation are now in the range of $150,000), increased funding for graduate medical education (GME) in primary care, and reallocation of GME training slots by specialty.

## 7. Address ethical issues in cancer care.

In our market-based system where the business model of care can trump the interests of patients, ethical considerations frequently become part of the equation in cancer care. We have already noted a number of examples of conflicts-of-interest among providers, researchers and facilities. In addition, of course, cancer as a life-threatening disease raises many bioethical questions for patients and their families as they work through their own decision-making. Advances in technology have brought controversy to many life-prolonging treatments, and both technical and non-technical judgments become important as patients deal with their own illness.

Many observers have called attention to the need for greater emphasis on the teaching and practice of bioethics in cancer care. These are some of the areas where improvements would be helpful:

- *Assure that newly diagnosed cancer patients are offered multidisciplinary advice on all of their treatment options.* This is frequently done through such means as Tumor Boards, which involve discussions with oncologists, radiation therapists and surgeons. But many patients are not given the opportunity to consider all of their options, and are encouraged to proceed with treatment with emphasis on only one of these modalities.

- *Increase patient participation in shared clinical decision-making whereby the individual patient's preferences and values can better inform choices among alternative treatments and outcomes.* Expand the use of decision aids to work through tradeoffs between benefits and harms of screening and treatment.

- *Help patients to interpret the statistics of their disease.* Stephen Jay Gould's experience is especially helpful in this regard. A renowned evolutionary biologist, paleontologist and educator at Harvard University, Gould faced the diagnosis of abdominal mesothelioma in 1982. When he was informed that the median survival time after diagnosis was only 8 months. After his initial treatment, he removed himself to the Harvard Library, read up on biostatistics, and became acquainted with "medians that are skewed to the right." He recognized the difference between mean survival (an overall average) and median survival (a different kind of halfway point, where patients surviving to the right (or beyond) the median may live for many years. Gould read further about his disease, decided that he had an excellent chance to live many more years since he was relatively young, the cancer was found early, and he had had good treatment. This gave him hope, he later wrote in an excellent essay *The Median Isn't the Message* (which should be required reading for all cancer patients). Though he died at 60 of another unrelated cancer, he had survived a remarkable 20 years following the onset of a disease with an initial prognosis of months.[40,41] Few patients have the background in statistics to ferret out what was for Gould a life-saving realization. Yet so many could use a more sophisticated understanding of what they face than what their doctors give them.

- *Strengthen counseling for patients and their families.* Patients need more help than they usually get in navigating the course of their illness from diagnosis through treatment, survival care, palliative and terminal care, if that becomes necessary. Longevity is often emphasized among treatment options regardless of quality of life along the way. The shift from cure or remission goals of treatment to palliative treatment is often delayed or not discussed, as is seen with many patients receiving chemotherapy in their last weeks or months of life. Whatever the circumstances and local resources, many disciplines can contribute to needed counseling, including physicians, nurses, social workers, and mental health professionals.

- *Address conflicts-of-interest in both clinical practice and research.* In the last 15 years, there has been an exponential growth in for-profit human experimentation companies (HECs), most of which operate outside academic medical centers. Colorado-based Coast Institutional Review Board, a for-profit ethics company, advertises on its Web site that it can save clients $6 million a day in guaranteed one-day turnaround time for Institutional Review Board approval of a research project. The FDA has recently ordered that company to suspend its use of expedited review procedures as potentially endangering the rights or welfare of human subjects.[42] Just recently coming to light, these HECs are only one example of conflicts of interest (COIs) which permeate the delivery of cancer care services. We described others in Chapter 6, such as over-utilization of imaging services, rebates for chemotherapy and anemia drugs, and self-referral by physicians to facilities in which they have an ownership stake. As we also saw, the world of cancer research is also fraught with many COIs throughout the research process, ranging from what subjects are addressed and the methods of study to how the results are interpreted and reported. Many of these COIs are now hidden to most outside observers, but moving toward a more accountable system under NHI will expose and reduce these kinds of problems.

## 8. Empower regulators to provide oversight and accountability of best products and practices.

Although health care takes up one-sixth of the nation's GDP, we still have no effective regulatory apparatus in place to assure cost-effectiveness of products or practices. Over the past three decades, market interests have lobbied successfully to maintain a deregulated system, as these two examples illustrate:

- The FDA, although charged with the responsibility to regulate drugs and medical devices, is dependent on industry through user fees for much of its budget, is understaffed and underfunded, cannot apply cost-effectiveness as a criterion for coverage decisions, has no authority to subpoena industry records to investigate suspected problems, cannot levy civil penalties for violations of its regulations, and lacks the authority to mandate drug recalls when not done voluntarily by drug manufacturers.[43] Medical device legislation in 2002 exempted many new devices from review and continues to apply a review criterion that only asks whether an applicant new device is equivalent to devices used before 1976.[44]

  MammoSite, a device developed to insert radioactive "seeds" after cancer breast surgery, illustrates the problems of lax review by the FDA. After a "quick-review" process, it was cleared by the FDA for use as an experimental treatment in 2002, without actual approval. It has been performed on about 45,000 women between 2002 and 2009, is still considered experimental, and it remains unproven that it works as well as conventional radiation treatment for breast cancer.[45] A 2009 GAO report concluded that the FDA should adopt a more stringent pre-market review process for high-risk medical devices.[46]

- Regulation of U.S. hospitals is similarly lax. When Medicare was enacted in 1965, oversight was delegated to the Joint Commission on the Accreditation of Healthcare Organizations

(JCAHO), a not-for-profit organization based in Oakbrook Terrace, Illinois. By means of periodic inspections of facilities, the JCAHO is tasked to monitor quality in 17,000 hospitals, nursing homes, and assisted-living facilities. However, its clout is limited by being dependent on income from facilities being inspected for much of its budget, understaffing, conflicts-of-interest, lack of transparency in its activities, and political interference in its efforts to downsize or shut down facilities with poor, even dangerous quality of care.[47,48]

Obviously, we need regulatory agencies that are non-partisan, well staffed and budgeted, free from political interference, with the mandate and authority to protect the public interest.

## Toward A Paradigm Shift In U.S. Health Care

The above eight-point plan is a coherent and interdependent vision for lasting health care reform. NHI is the essential underpinning, but the other seven directions are also vitally needed. As examples, NHI can assure affordable access to cancer care, but we need that care to be scientifically sound and state of the art. We need a system within which waste, inappropriate and unnecessary care are not rewarded. So that reimbursement reform is therefore mandatory (which in turn can start to encourage return of young physicians to primary care and other critical shortage fields). So each of these eight directions adds to the impact of the others, and without all eight, meaningful reform becomes less likely.

It is also important to note that the above eight-point plan, if implemented, will represent a much needed and long overdue paradigm shift. It will narrow the gap in access, quality and equity of health care between this country and other advanced countries around the world. What do we mean by this paradigm shift?

Over time, a five-way shift will have to occur if real health care reform is to take place and the American Cancer Society's goal of 4 As is to be achieved:

1. Health care is a right, not a privilege.
2. Access is based on medical need, not ability to pay.
3. System is redesigned primarily for patients, not providers and markets.
4. In a not-for-profit system, health care is not just another commodity for sale on an open market.
5. The interests of society receive increased weight in order to assure that the best possible care, within limited resources, is available for all Americans, not just the more affluent.

Given the gravity of personal hardship of millions of Americans in dealing with a failing health care system during bad economic times, this kind of paradigm shift is arguably a moral, economic and social imperative. This shift will involve public financing of a private delivery system. Physicians, other health care professionals and facilities will compete the old-fashioned way – by availability, quality, and effectiveness of care. All patients will pay into the system through taxes, all will have the dignity of paying patients, and many will fare better than they now do in our current system.

The new system will not be perfect – there is no such thing. But our present system is failing despite all incremental efforts over the years to fix it. A new system reformed along the above lines fits our espoused American ideals of hard work, equal opportunity, and egalitarianism. Table 11.2 summarizes alternative futures with or without this paradigm shift.

## So What Will Happen?

Lives hang in the balance on the answer to this question. The future down our current path is crystal clear – and devastating. Deregulated markets and the corrosive effects of profits over service over many years have brought U.S. health care to a crisis point. Because of soaring costs, patients with cancer are finding effective care increasingly unaffordable. Health care has entered a perfect storm, and it is certain to get much worse without real reform. Our primary care infrastructure is collapsing, ERs are overwhelmed, the ranks of the unemployed are rising quickly, adding to the numbers of uninsured. The economy has tanked, the federal deficit is massive, many states are forced to cut Medicaid to the bone, and our presumed safety net is falling apart.

TABLE 11.2

# Alternate Futures Based on Paradigm

| Financing | Single-payer | Multi-payer |
|---|---|---|
| **Access** | Universal access, one-tier | Decreasing access, multi-tier |
| **Costs** | Manageable | Uncontrolled inflation |
| **System quality** | Improved | Degraded |
| **Health disparities** | Diminished | Aggravated |
| **Equity** | Improved | Worse |
| **System efficiency** | Improved | Decreased |
| **Bureaucracy** | Simplified | Increased and more fragmented |
| **Sustainability** | Improved | Imploding on itself |
| **Social fabric** | Strengthened | Further frayed |
| **U.S. workforce** | More competitive | Less competitive |
| **Population health** | Improved | Declining |
| **Public satisfaction** | Increased | Decreased |

Meanwhile, market stakeholders increase their efforts to maintain the status quo. The private insurance industry calls for the government to change tax policy and keep the subsidies flowing so that insurers can continue to rake off their profits from the system while offloading sicker and lower-income patients onto public programs. AARP, beholden

## FIGURE 11.1

# Fundraising by U.S. Senators for the 2003-2008 Election Cycle

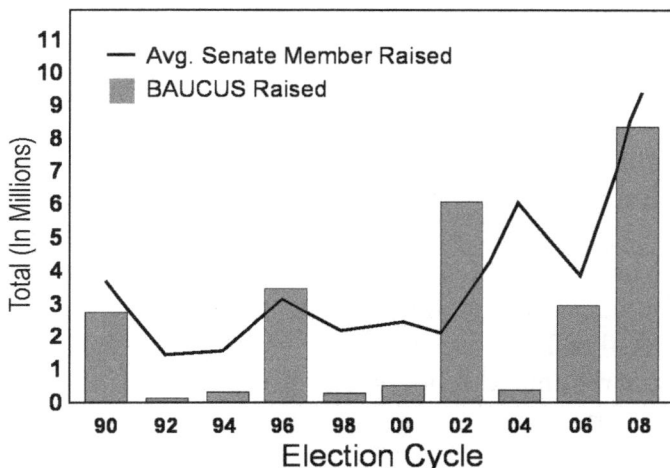

Source: OpenSecrets.org. Senator Max Baucus. Cycle Fundraising, 2003-2008. March 6, 2009. Accessed on http://www.opensecrets.org/politicians/summary. php?cid=N000046.

as it is to UnitedHealth , the nation's second largest health insurer, for revenues from its endorsed products, postures about "reform" that would maintain that industry in place. Conflicts of interest are widespread among our political leaders, and the revolving door moves freely between government, industry, and the K Street lobbying nexus.

Campaign contributions, as the nectar of politics, continue to have an enormous influence over policymaking, though this is typically denied by those involved. Figure 11.1, based on figures from the Center for Responsive Politics, shows how much money was raised by U.S. senators during the 2003 to 2008 election cycle, including that raised by Senator Baucus, the Chairman of the Senate Finance Committee. Baucus raised more than $11 million over those 5 years, including more than half a million dollars from each of three industries – insurance, pharmaceuticals/health care products, and health professionals.[49] When asked about single-payer NHI during a 2009 interview with *Time Magazine's* Karen Tumulty, he rejected it out of hand in no uncertain terms: "We are not Europe. We are not Canada. We are America. This is not a single pay country."[50] Is it any wonder that he has worked so hard to keep single-payer off the table of possible reform alternatives?

The political influence of lobbyists is a major impediment to health care reform. Over the last 40 years lobbying has grown from a small group of lawyers and influence peddlers to a multi-billion dollar industry involving thousands of people, including almost 200 ex-senators and ex-House members from both parties.[51] They are supported, of course, by corporate interests trying to preserve the status quo of our market-based system. In the first weeks of the new Congress and Administration in 2009, lobbyists were actively trying to shoot down or minimize attempted reforms. Here are two examples:

- The drug and medical device industries opposed the use of cost-effectiveness research as a guide to policy-making by any new Clinical Effectiveness agency as "the first step toward government rationing." A new coalition was formed, deceptively called the Partnership to Improve Patient Care, which includes the lobbying arms of the drug, biotechnology, and medical device industries, together with patient advocacy groups and some medical professional societies.[52]
- On the day after President Obama's first address to Congress, Richard Scott, former CEO of HCA, Inc., the nation's largest for-profit hospital chain, announced a $20 million campaign to pressure members of Congress to base future health care legislation on free-market principles. This effort also included a new coalition, again with a misleading name: Conservatives for Patients' Rights.[53]

The battle in 2009-2010 over health care reform showed the political power and influence of corporate money over politicians on both sides of the aisle. Single payer was kept off the table, and the sharpest debate focused on the so-called public option as the maximal possible insurance reform. It was soon killed in the political crossfire. Even if a public option had survived to be included in the Affordable Care Act, it would not have worked. For starters, it would have cost much more right off the bat, foregoing 84 percent of cost savings that would be achieved under single-payer NHI. Figure 11.2 shows how administrative costs would have compared if one-half of the privately insured switched over to the public plan option.[54] The public option would have further fragmented the system, still not provide universal access, not contain costs, and fail to stabilize the system. It would have given the illusion of reform but delayed real reform for more years as the situation becomes worse. By the time the Affordable Care Act was finally passed in 2010, the lobbying industry had reaped its own bonanza—some 1,750 organizations and businesses had hired 4,525 lobbyists—eight for every member of Congress, at a cost of $1.2 billion.[55]

## FIGURE 11.2

# Administrative Costs:
## Single-Payer vs. Public Plan Option

**Public Plan Option Saves Little Even if Half of Previously Insured Switch**

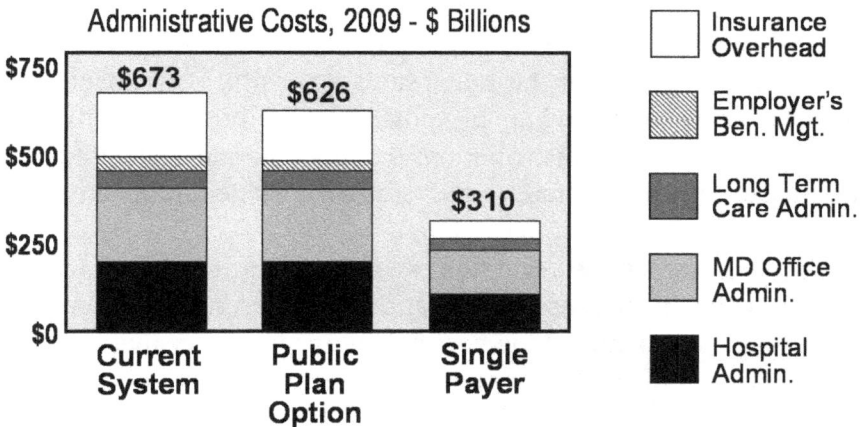

Source: Woolhandler S, Campbell T, Himmelstein DU. Costs of health care administration in the United States and Canada. *N Engl J Med* 349: 768, 2003, with calculations updated to 2009. Reprinted with permission.

It is therefore not surprising that politicians on both sides of the aisle still seem to think that incremental changes in a private-public financing system can resolve our crisis in costs, access, and quality of care. And even when confronted about the single-payer option, most still try to keep it off the table, fearing to take on the insurance industry and other corporate stakeholders in the medical-industrial complex.

While many of our legislators dare not deal with the merits of single-payer, they posture as reformers with such small steps as expanding SCHIP, expanding eligibility for COBRA benefits, or trying other ways to "regulate" private insurers. But, as we have seen, all of these attempts will fail because they don't address the core problems – market failure while retaining an obsolete insurance industry, which would already be dead without government subsidies.

Recall from Chapter 1 that the first cancer hospital in the world, in Reims, France, was forced to close because of the public's fear of contagion. Cancer was thought to be spread by parasites. *Today, we have blinders on when we do not see the market failure all around us.*

We should be able to expect that all reform alternatives be fairly evaluated and objectively compared on such measures as comparative costs and how well they will improve access, quality and equity of U.S. health care. However, that is not the way our political process works. We saw in Chapter 9 how single-payer NHI wins hands down on all these measures against private financing. The facts are quite clear, but still most of our politicians, conflicted as they are by large contributions from corporate stakeholders, continue to deny market failure and refuse to consider the advantages of single-payer.

As the deepening recession keeps adding to the number of uninsured and underinsured, the health care crisis only gets worse. The many system problems of the health insurance industry that have been described here only add to the pain and misery of millions of Americans. Indeed, the health insurance industry itself is a big part of the problem, and certainly not part of the solution. Even as the industry keeps raising its premiums (with declining enrollments), it can look ahead to as many as 32 million new enrollees (many through government subsidies), if the Affordable Care Act is not repealed or underfunded after the 2012 elections. So Wall Street and private health insurers are still happy. UnitedHealth Group, the largest insurer in terms of revenue and market value, saw its stock prices jump to a 52-week high within a day after reporting a 13 percent increase in profits for the first quarter of 2011; the five other largest insurers had similar gains the next day. [56]

Despite the resounding rhetoric to the contrary, our health care system cannot be fixed through more political compromises by centrists. Given the nature of politics in this country and the political power of corporate stakeholders, a bipartisan solution is not likely, and will only yield more compromises that perpetuate the status quo. We need to remember that passage of Medicare and Medicaid in the 1960s was a bitter partisan fight down to the wire. In the final votes in Congress, 68 Republicans and 48 Democrats voted against them in the House, with 7 Democrats and 17 Republicans also doing so in the Senate.[57]

Is there any room for optimism? In the longer run, for sure, because the kinds of directions in the above eight-point plan will inevitably be necessary. Health professionals are increasingly frustrated with current market bureaucracies; three of five U.S. physicians now support NHI.[58] Organized labor is becoming energized about the need for NHI, and business may not be far behind as economic pressures mount. Public support for NHI will likely get stronger as our system further implodes. The electorate is changing, with younger adults in the Millennial Generation taking more progressive views on economic issues. "Millennials" have become the largest generation in size, already 80 to 95 million strong, with three in five supporting NHI and nearly nine in ten believing that the government should spend more on health care even if a tax increase becomes necessary.[59] And the Baby Boomer generation is being hit by costs of their own care, as well as that of their parents, at a time when their savings have disappeared, their 401(k)s have evaporated, and their planned retirements delayed.

But reform will ultimately require a broad political movement forcing our politicians to avoid political compromises that will guarantee policy failure. The Occupy Wall Street movement spreading across the country is likely to start creating a widespread political movement against the power of Wall Street and the 1 percent. It has already made a big difference, as described in an important *Truthout* article in November 2011 *Ten Ways the Occupy Movement Changes Everything*. These are some of the ways: [60]

• It names the source of the crisis as—"The problems of the 99 percent are caused in large part by Wall

Street greed, perverse financial incentives, and a corporate takeover of the political system."

• It sets a new standard for public debate: those advocating policies and proposals must now demonstrate that their ideas will benefit the 99 percent.

• It is a movement, not a list of demands. The call is for deep change, not temporary fixes and single-issue reforms.

We can hope that health care reform will be caught up in a new era of progressive reforms that could also include new efforts to deal with unemployment, homelessness, and threats to Medicare and Social Security. Robert Reich, former Secretary of Labor in the Clinton administration and Professor of Public Policy at the University of California Berkeley, gives us this encouraging overview:

"The great arc of American history reveals an unmistakable pattern. Whenever privilege and power conspire to pull us backward, the nation eventually rallies and moves forward. . . . Look at the progressive reforms between 1900 and 1916; the New Deal of the 1930s; the Civil Rights struggle of the 1950s and 1960s; the widening opportunities for women, minorities, people with disabilities, and gays; and the environmental reforms of the 1970s.

In each of these eras, regressive forces reignited the progressive ideals on which America is built. The result was fundamental reform. Perhaps this is what's beginning to happen again across America."[61]

We are all patients at one time or another. Many of us are cancer patients, or have a family member, neighbor or close friend with cancer. We are all in the same boat. None of us want to deal with cancer, but one way or another, all of us will have to. At that point, there is a real question whether or not effective care will be affordable and accessible to us unless real system reform is tackled soon.

We can all play an activist role, wherever we live, in advocating for health care reform. Appendix 4 lists organizations by state that would welcome your involvement. It also provides information on how grassroots groups can join a new national single-payer alliance, the Leadership Conference for Guaranteed Health Care.

We can take inspiration for the task ahead from these words by Dr. Martin Luther King, Jr.:

"Of all the forms of inequality, injustice in health care is the most shocking and most inhuman... Although social change cannot come overnight, we must always work as though it were a possibility in the morning."

It all comes down to these final questions. Are we in America so cruel as to deny our fellow Americans the opportunity to avoid cancer or get well if they get it? Is cancer care only for the more affluent among us? Are we the civilized and caring society we claim to be? The time to answer these questions is upon us. Will we?

# References:

1.  Hayek FA, as quoted in a condensed version in the April, 1945 edition of *Reader's Digest.*
2.  Adopted by the General Assembly on December 10, 1948. Printed in: von Munch I, Buske, A (eds), International Law: the Essential Treaties and Other Relevant documents. 1985 435ff.
3.  Lakoff, G, Haas E, Smith GW, et al. The Logic of the Health Care Debate. Berkeley, CA: A Rockridge Institute Report. October 15, 2007. (available at http://www.rockridgeinstitute.org/.
4.  McCanne D. Quote of the Day on December 31, 2008 (don@mccanne.org) commenting on article by Morrisey, M A, Cawley, J. Health economists' views of health policy. *Journal of Health Politics, Policy and Law*, August, 2008.
5.  Geyman JP. *Do Not Resuscitate: Why the Health Insurance Industry Is Dying, and How We Must Replace It.* Monroe, ME. Common Courage Press, 2008: p 186.
6.  Seager A. Development: U.S. fails to measure up on "human index". *The Guardian*, July 17, 2008.
7.  Lewis K. Testimony before the Joint Economic Committee, July 23, 2008; available at http://jec.senate.gov/index.efm?FuseAction=Hearings. HearingsCalendar&contentrecord      _id=4b4275bc-d7b2-8563-4faf-a21bf-4898ba4.
8.  Editorial. Health care by loopholes. *AARP Bulletin* 48 (3): 3, 2007.
9.  Gross D. National health care? We're halfway there. *New York Times*, December 3, 2006.
10. DrSteveB. AHIP endorses mandates: universal health or bailout boondoggle? *Daily Kos* November 20, 2008.
11. Boylan LS. Single-payer: mainstream and "shovel ready". Letter to Editor, *The New Yorker*, January 30, 2009.
12. Kaiser Daily Health Policy Report, August 4, 2008.
13. MedPAC, A Data Book: Healthcare Spending and the Medicare Program, 2008.
14. Dentzer S. The imaging boom. *Health Aff (Millwood)* 27 (6): 1466. 2008.
15. Rabin RC. With rise in radiation exposure, experts urge caution on tests. *New York Times,* June 19, 2007.
16. Neumann PJ, Kumae MS, Palmer JA. Medicare's national coverage decisions for technologies, 1999-2007, *Health Aff (Millwood)* 27 (6): 1620-31, 2008.

17. Orszag PR. Growth in Health Care Costs. CBO Testimony before the Committee on the Budget, United States Senate, Congressional Budget Office, January 31, 2008.
18. Buxton MJ. Economic evaluation and decision making in the U K. *Pharmacoeconomics* 24: 1133-42, 2008.
19. Laupacis A. Economic evaluations in the Canadian common drug review. *Pharmacoeconomics* 24: 1157-62, 2006.
20. Moses H, Dorsey ER, Mathesen DHM, et al. Financial anatomy of biomedical research. *JAMA* 294 (11): 1333-42, 2005.
21. Baker D. The benefits and savings from publicly funded clinical trials of prescription drugs. *Intl. J Health Services* 38 (4): 731-50. 2008.
22. Thornton M. The next front in the war on cancer. Op-Ed. *Wall Street Journal*, February 27, 2009: A17.
23. Kolata G. New arena for testing of drugs: real world. *New York Times*, November 25, 2008: D1.
24. Pinkowish MD. Recruitment to breast cancer clinical trials: What makes a difference? *CA: A Cancer Journal for Clinicians* 59 (1): 1-2, 2009.
25. Breaking through the myths: Cancer clinical trials may not be what you thought. *CURE* 7 (5), 2008.
26. Choudry NK, Stelfox HT, Detsky AS. Relationships between authors of clinical practice guidelines and the pharmaceutical industry. *JAMA* 287 (5): 612-7, 2002.
27. NCCN. Web site of the National Comprehensive Cancer Network. http://www.nccn.org/ ,accessed February 9, 2009.
28. Wilson, D. Study finds conflicts among panels' doctors. *New York Times*, March 29, 2011: B3.
29. Bellizzi KM, Mustian KM, Bowen DJ, et al. Aging in the context of cancer prevention and control: Perspectives from behavioral medicine. *CANCER* 113 (12 Suppl): 3479-83, December 15, 2008, as quoted in Science Daily , December 13, 2008.
30. Himmelstein DU, Woolhandler S. The corporate compromise: A Marxist view of health policy. *Monthly Review* (May 14): 20-22, 1990.
31. Bach PB. Paying doctors to ignore patients. *New York Times*, July 24, 2008: A23.
32. Relman AS. *A Second Opinion: Rescuing America's Health Care.* New York. Public Affairs, 2008, p 139.
33. ACP. The impending collapse of primary care medicine and its implications for the state of the nation's health care. Washington, DC. American College of Physicians, January 30, 2006. Accessed August 10, 2006 at http://www.acponline.org/hpp/statehc06 1pdf.
34. Committee on the Future of Health Care Workforce for Older Americans. Retooling for an aging America: building the health care workforce. Washington, DC: National Academies Press, 2008.
35. Erikson C, Salsberg E, Forte G, et al. Future supply and demand of oncologists: Challenges to assuring access to oncology services. *J Oncol Pract* 3: 79-86, 2007.

36. Dorsey ER, Jarjoura D, Rutecki GW. The influence of controllable lifestyles and sex on the specialty choices of graduating medical students, 1996-2003, *Acad Med* 80: 791-6, 2005.

37. Seward ZM. Doctor shortage hurts a coverage-for-all plan. *Wall Street Journal*, July 25, 2007: B1.

38. Forrest CB. Strengthening primary care to bolster the health care safety net. *JAMA* 295 (9):1062-4, 2006.

39. Earle CC, Neville BA. Under use of necessary care among cancer survivors. *Cancer* 101 (8): 1712-19, 2004.

40. Yoon CK. Stephen Jay Gould, 60, is dead; enlivened evolutionary theory. *New York Times*, May 21, 2002.

41. CancerGuide: Statistics. Gould SJ. The Median Isn't the Message. Available on http://www.cancerguide.org/median_not_msg.html, accessed on November, 17, 2008.

42. Outrage of the Month. Human experimentation and speedy for-profit ethical review boards. Washington, DC. Public Citizen *Research Group, Health Letter* 24 (6): 9-10, 2008.

43. Siegelman D. Unsafe drugs: Congressional silence is deadly. *Public Citizen Research Group, Health Letter* 18: 1, 2002.

44. Deyo RA, Patrick DL. Hope or Hype: The Obsession with Medical Advances and the High Cost of False Promises. New York. American Management Association, 2005, p265.

45. Abelson R. Treatment, quickly vetted, is offered to cancer patients. *New York Times*, October 27, 2009: A1.

46. GAO. Medical Devices. FDA should take steps to ensure that high-risk device types are approved through the most stringent premarket review process. Washington, DC. United States Government Accountability Office, January, 2009.

47. Gaul GM. Medicare's oversight gap: Accreditors are blamed for overlooking problems, and for conflicts of interest. *Washington Post National Weekly Edition*, April 8-14, 2005: 8-9.

48. Berenson A. Weak patchwork of oversight lets bad hospitals stay open. *New York Times,* December 8, 2008: A1.

49. OpenSecrets.org. Senator Max Baucus. Cycle Fundraising, 2003-2008. March 6, 2009. Accessed on http://www.opensecrets.org/politicians/summary. php?cid=N000046...

50. Baucus M, as quoted in interview with Karen Tumulty from Time Magazine in a Health Care Reform Newsmaker Series, March 3, 2009. Kaiser Family Foundation.

51. Kaiser RG. Special interests: Obama's most ambitious promise may be the one to curb K Street lobbyists. *The Washington Post National Weekly Edition,* February 9-15, 2009, p 27.

52. Mundy A. Drug makers fight stimulus provision. *Wall Street Journal*, February 10, 2009: A4.

53. Mullins B, Kilman S. Lobbyists line up to torpedo speech proposals. *Wall Street Journal*, February 26, 2009: A4.

54. Woolhandler S, Campbell T, Himmelstein DU. Costs of health care administration in the United States and Canada. *N Engl J Med* 349: 768, 2003, with calculations updated to 2009.

55. Center for Public Integrity, as cited by Moyers, B, Winship, M. The unbearable lightness of reform. *Truthout*, March 27, 2011.

56. Potter, W. Health insurance execs making more than ever before. *Huffpost Business*, April 25, 2011.

57. Legislative History. H.R. 6675, The Social Security Amendments of 1965. Social Security Online.

58. Carroll AE, Ackermann RT. Support for national health insurance among U.S. physicians: Five years later. *Ann Intern Med* 148: 566-7, 2008. .

59. Madland D, Logan A. The progressive generation: how young adults think about the economy.
    Center for American Progress, May 6, 2008.

60. van Gelder, S, Korten, D, Piersanti, S. Ten Ways the Occupy Movement Changes Everything. *Truthout*, November 10, 2011.

61. Reich, RB. Right wing radicals awaken progressive movement. *The Progressive Populist*, November 15, 2011, p. 13.

# AFTERWORD

# The Torch is in Your Hands:
# A Cross-Generational Message to Baby Boomers

The Torch is in Your Hands:
A Cross-Generational Message to Baby Boomers

Your generation has been given a deadly diagnosis: National health insurance is not possible. You've been living with this news for some time as most politicians say that it's "not politically feasible." And you've been given all kinds of palliative care, from privatization of Medicare to health insurance for some children to other assurances that the market will fix our problems, if you will just be patient, with a few modest reforms. But you are becoming financially exhausted and know that the system is getting sicker every day. Yet the prescription never changes – have faith in the market.

Here is what I know about you, the Baby Boomer generation:

First, your parents have passed onto you a predisposition for taking on big challenges. Your parents won World War II, then brought on reforms of the 1960s and landed a man on the moon. You have inherited their strength, and have a keen sense of both sacrifice and justice – sacrifice by being willing to fight in Vietnam and justice in protesting against the war until you forced it to end.

Yours is a generation of firsts. You have founded many types of businesses, from personal computing to an entire entrepreneurial ecosystem on the Internet. You elected our first African-American president. You are the generation who can bring about the justice that the majority of Americans have been seeking for more than 50 years.

My prescription is simple: Take action daily as needed.

In becoming an activist for health care reform, you have a wide range of tools at your disposal. Which ones are best for you depends on your own strengths. Will it be letter writing? Organizing demonstrations? Mounting legal challenges? Creating a new political social network on the Web? From history you can see that everyday actions can be surprisingly effective. Who would have thought that sitting down in a bus would mark a pivotal moment in the civil rights movement? No doubt the struggle to make essential health care available to all Americans will take its surprising turns as well. As Thomas Jefferson once wrote in a letter to James Madison: "A little rebellion now and then is a good thing, and as necessary in the political world as storms are in the physical..."

Whether you have cancer or you don't, whether you get cancer or you don't, as a member of the Baby Boomer generation, you are moving through the prime of your life. You have reached the point, or will soon reach it, where you ask the question, what legacy will I leave behind? Now is the time to start shaping your answer.

More than two millennia ago, Euripides lamented:

"We know the good, we apprehend it clearly, but we cannot bring it to achievement."

If ever there was a generation who could prove Euripides wrong, who could bring about the social justice that so many Americans clearly apprehend, your generation is it. Your time has come. We need your drive, creative energy, and sense of fair play. You can bring justice in health care, as our common birthright, for yourselves, your children, and generations to follow.

Take the torch. Accept the challenge. Many will help you. You can do it!

# APPENDIX 1

# Glossary

**Adjuvant Therapy:** Treatment used in addition to the main cancer treatment, often referring to other treatments after surgery.[1]

**Adverse Selection:** This occurs when lower-risk individuals are split off by insurers from a larger risk pool in order to minimize their financial risk and increase these profits. The smaller risk pool of higher-risk individuals that results requires higher costs of treatment. Adverse selection is the Achilles' heel of capitation, since for-profit HMOs and some physicians are often tempted to selectively care for healthier patients.[2]

**Agency for Healthcare Research and Quality (AHRQ):** This federal agency was established by Congress in 1989 as the Agency for Health Care Policy and Research (AHCPR). Since then, its name has been changed, but its continuing activities include development of clinical practice guidelines, promotion of evidence-based medicine, reduction of medical errors, and expansion of research on the cost, utilization, and outcomes of health care.[2]

**America's Health Insurance Plans (AHIP):** This is a national trade group representing about 1,300 member private insurance companies which provide coverage to about 200 million Americans. It was formed in 2003 by the merger of the American Association of Health Plans (AAHP) and the Health Insurance Association of America (HIAA).[2]

**Association Health Plans (AHPs):** These are plans established by private insurers in order to better market their policies across state lines. AHPs are exempt from state rate-setting regulations in many states. Insurers claim that AHPs can make insurance more affordable for smaller employers while critics argue that AHPs allow insurers more latitude to "cherry pick" the market without assurances of adequate coverage.[2]

**Capitation:** A method of payment for patient care services used by managed care organizations, such as health maintenance organizations (HMOs), to reimburse providers under contractual agreements. Payment rates are set in advance, and are paid monthly or annually regardless of what services are actually provided to covered patients.[2]

**Carrier**: Private insurers which contract with Medicare to administer supplementary health insurance under Part B of Medicare. In the earlier years,

Blue Shield held most of these contracts for physician services. Today's decentralized market has many commercial insurers involved as carriers.[2]

**Center for Medicare and Medicaid Services (CMS):** The federal agency which administers the Medicare program and works with the states to administer Medicaid, the State Children's Health Insurance Program (SCHIP), and health insurance portability standards. CMS accounts for 20% of the federal government's budget. In FY 2005, this amounted to about $519 billion, with nearly two-thirds of that spent on Medicare.[2]

**COBRA (The Consolidated Omnibus Budget Reconciliation Act of 1985):** This is the mechanism by which people who lose or change jobs which provide employer-based health insurance may regain insurance through the individual market if they can afford the premiums. Under COBRA, insurers and health plans are required to continue their previous coverage for at least 18 months.[2]

**Co-Insurance:** This refers to the percentage of health care costs which are not covered by insurance and which the individual must pay. Many health insurance plans cover 80% of the costs of hospital and physician care, leaving 20% to be "self-insured" by patients receiving these services.[2]

**Community Health Centers (CHCs):** These are safety net facilities and primary care practices which are intended to serve their communities regardless of ability to pay. Through federal funding and smaller public and private grants, CHCs seek to improve the health status of all members of the community, many of whom are uninsured. There are more than 1,000 CHCs located in underserved communities across the country. [2]

**Community Rating:** A method for setting premiums for health insurance which is based on the average cost of health care for the covered population in a geographic area. This method shares risk across all covered individuals, whether sick or well, so that the healthy help to subsidize the care of the sick who otherwise may not be able to afford coverage on their own. As a then not-for-profit insurer, Blue Cross pioneered this method in the 1930s, but it was abandoned by most commercial insurers after the 1960s, as experience rating spread throughout the industry.[2]

**Co-Morbidity:** The presence of other medical conditions that may be relevant to a patient's outcome.[3]

**Consumer-Directed Health Care (CDHC):** A strategy to contain health care costs by shifting more responsibility to consumers in choosing and paying for their own health care. Currently popular with conservatives and many moderates in government, the consumer-choice theory of cost containment assumes that there is a free market in health care, that consumers can be well informed about their choices, and that they will be more prudent in their health care decisions by taking more responsibility to pay for their costs.[2]

**Cost Effectiveness:** When applied to health care, this concept attempts to estimate the value for expenditures on procedures or services that is returned to patients. Value may include longer life, better quality of life, or both. This is a complex but important area of study if affordable care of good quality is to be made available to broad populations. Cost-effectiveness analysis (CEA) is the technique used to measure costs and efficacy of alternative treatments in order to estimate their economic value, which then are typically measured in quality-adjusted life years (QALYs).[2]

**Co-Payment:** Flat fee charged directly to patients whenever they seek health care services or drug prescriptions regardless of their insurance coverage. As today's trend toward consumer-directed health care gains momentum, co-payments are increasing across the health care marketplace to the point of becoming a financial barrier to care for many lower-income people.[2]

**Cost-Sharing:** This term refers to requirements that patients pay directly out-of-pocket for some portion of their health care costs. The level of cost-sharing varies from one health plan to another. Although intended by insurers and many policy makers to help control the costs of health care, cost-sharing has a serious downside of discouraging many people from gaining access to necessary health care.[2]

**Death Spiral:** This term is used to describe the progressive effects of adverse selection in shrinking a risk pool into a smaller population of high-risk individuals requiring expensive care. For example, as a result of "cream-skimming" by for-profit private health plans, public programs such as Medicare are placed at risk because of reduced cross subsidies from the healthy to the sick.[2]

**Deductible:** Out-of-pocket costs which patients must pay before their insurance coverage kicks in for subsequent costs. This amount is required to be met each year. As policy-makers and health plans pursue the model of consumer-directed health care, deductibles and co-payment requirements of cost-sharing are increasing each year.[2]

**Defined Benefits:** This term is applied when an insurance program offers a pre-determined set of benefits to all enrollees. The Medicare program is such an example, with covered benefits authorized by law.[2]

**Defined Contributions:** This is the polar opposite of defined benefits. In this instance, a fixed set of benefits is not provided by the insurer, whether public or private. Instead, a defined contribution is made toward the costs of coverage (e.g., by an employer or perhaps by Medicare if further privatization "reforms" are enacted) (see also Premium Support).[2]

**Disease Management:** This is a new buzzword being hailed by many policy makers and legislators for its potential to rein in health care costs and improve the quality of care for chronic diseases such as diabetes. While effective primary care team-based disease management programs have been pioneered by not-for-profit organizations such as Group Health Cooperative and Kaiser Permanente for some years, a for-profit commercial DM industry has emerged, started by the drug industry during the 1990s, which attempts to provide patient education and improved patient self-management, mostly through nurses in distant call centers without integration with primary care.[2]

**Distributive Justice:** When used in health care, this term connotes a principle of fairness whereby health care is considered a right that should be shared within a society on the basis of need. The countervailing view held by proponents of an open market is that health care is a privilege that should be allocated by ability to pay. With an emphasis on markets, the U.S. is atypical from almost all other industrialized countries around the world where distributive justice is the dominant ethic underlying various systems of social health insurance.[2]

**Doughnut Hole Coverage:** This is the gap between partial coverage (75%) and catastrophic coverage (95%) of the costs of prescription drugs provided to Medicare beneficiaries through the Part D Prescription Drug Benefit. The Medicare legislation of 2003 (MMA) initially set the "doughnut hole between $2,250 and $5,100 annual drug costs (a $2,850 gap) within which Medicare beneficiaries are responsible to pay these costs out-of-pocket.[2]

**Effectiveness:** The ability of an intervention to achieve the desired results under usual conditions.[4]

**Employer-Based Insurance:** A voluntary system established during the wartime economy of the 1940s whereby many employers have provided health insurance overage to their employees. Today, that system is unraveling steadily, now covering only about two-thirds of the non-elderly workforce and with many employers shifting to a defined contribution approach toward their employees' insurance costs.[2]

**Employer-Mandate:** A policy considered in some states whereby all employers would be required to provide health insurance for their employees. Such a policy is usually opposed by small business, fearing costs that could put them out of business.[2]

**Experience Rating:** This is the current norm in U.S. health insurance markets, as opposed to the community rating tradition originally established by Blue Cross in the 1930s. Under experience rating, insurers avoid high-risk individuals and groups and increase premiums based upon illnesses experienced by enrollees. Experience rating weakens the ability of health insurance to share risk across a large risk pool of healthy and sick individuals. [2]

**Favorable Risk Selection:** This is the process by which insurers screen potential enrollees according to health status, avoiding higher-risk sick individuals and groups in favor of healthier enrollees requiring less costly care (i.e., the opposite of adverse selection).[2]

**Fee-for-Service (FFS):** A common method of reimbursement for health services provided, such as by visit, procedure, laboratory test or imaging study. Fees are often based on a fixed fee schedule or on more complex relative value scales.[2]

**Fiscal Intermediary:** Private insurers which contract with Medicare to administer hospitalization insurance under Part A of Medicare. Blue Cross has held most of these contracts over the years. In this capacity, insurers are empowered to make coverage and reimbursement decisions and to provide related administrative services.[2]

**Formulary:** Lists of drugs updated at regular intervals, which can be prescribed by physicians for enrollees in specific programs. Formularies have been developed by health plans in recent years as a means of containing escalating drug spending. Formulary development is a contentious area, with the pharmaceutical industry arguing for wider coverage lists while health plans strive to balance cost, efficacy and safety issues against patients' access to medically necessary medications.[2]

**Geographic Variation:** This term is used to describe wide variations from one part of the country to another in practice patterns and services provided to Medicare beneficiaries. Regional and small area variations date back to the origins of the program, including marked differences in utilization of services as well as coverage and reimbursement policies.[2]

**Generic Drugs:** Drugs which are essentially the same as their brand-name counterparts, but whose patents have expired. They are generally considerably less expensive than their brand-name equivalents.[2]

**Grade:** the grade of a tumor depends on how abnormal the cancer cells look under a microscope and how quickly the tumor is likely to grow and spread; grading systems vary from one cancer to another.[6]

**Group Market:** The private health insurance market is split into two distinct parts – group and individual markets. Group markets involve employer-based insurance, further divided into large groups and small groups. Since each state has its own regulations for the insurance industry, the overall insurance market is divided into 150 different state-level markets.[2]

**Guaranteed Issue:** Typically opposed by the private insurance industry because of the potential for adverse selection, some states require insurers to provide coverage to all comers, an open-enrollment policy.[2]

**Health Care Financing Administration (HCFA):** As part of the Department of Health and Human Services (DHHS), HCFA was created in 1977. It administered Medicare and Medicaid for many years until reconstituted in 2001 as the Center for Medicare and Medicaid Services (CMS).[2]

**Health Maintenance Organization (HMO):** HMOs are organizations which provide a broad range of services, coordinated by primary care physicians on a prepaid basis for enrollees. First authorized by federal legislation in 1973, HMOs have developed since the 1980s to now cover about 80 million Americans. About two-thirds of HMOs are for-profit, such as Humana, while the rest are not-for-profit, such as Kaiser Permanente and Group Health of Puget Sound. HMOs vary organizationally from staff models, where physicians are salaried and work only with that HMO (e.g., Kaiser and Group Health) to looser structures, such as independent practice associations (IPAs), where physicians in independent practices contract with an HMO to provide care for enrollees and are reimbursed on a capitation basis. Though it has become an imprecise term over the years, "managed care" encompasses these variations within an overall pattern of prepaid medical care.[2]

**Health Savings Account (HSA):** As part of the current trend toward consumer-directed health care, health savings accounts shift more financial responsibility to consumers for the costs of their health care decisions. HSAs were authorized under the Medicare Prescription Drug, Improvement, and Modernization Act of 2003 (MMA). Employer and employee contributions are tax-free when accompanied by high deductible insurance policies. While providing new investment opportunities for healthy individuals, HSAs provide little financial protection against the costs of serious illness.[2]

**High-Deductible Health Insurance Plans (HDHI):** As part of the present trend toward "consumer-directed" health care, many private insurers are offering policies with high cost-sharing requirements, including annual deductibles up to $10,000. These policies are typically associated with health savings accounts (HSAs) and provide little coverage or security for people experiencing significant medical expenses.[2]

**High-Risk Pool:** With the intent to help people who have been denied coverage in the individual market to gain coverage by pooling risk with others facing the same problem, about 30 states have established high-risk pools supported by both federal and state funding. To date, however, these high-risk pools have had little success in reducing the numbers of uninsured, and their limited coverage comes with high premiums.[2]

**Incidence:** Refers to the number of new cases of a given disease within a given time.[4]

**Individual Market:** Compared to employer-sponsored health insurance covering groups of employees, the individual market is relatively small, covering only 17 million non-elderly Americans. Many applicants are denied coverage in the individual market. For those who qualify, premiums are higher and coverage less secure.[4]

**Lead-Time Bias:** Apparent lengthening of survival due to earlier diagnosis in the course of disease but without any actual prolongation of life.[4]
**Length Bias:** Bias due to the tendency of screening tests to detect a larger number of cases of slowly progressing disease and miss aggressive disease due to its rapid progression.[4]

**Limited-Benefit Plan:** These are policies being marketed by private insurers to employers and healthier people with restricted benefits and annual caps as low as $1,000 to $2,500.[2]

**Managed Care:** Although this term has often become ambiguous and unclear in common usage, it expresses a new relationship between purchasers, insurers and providers of care. To a variable extent, organizations that pay for patient care have also taken on the role of making decisions about patient care management. In practice, however, "managed care" is often more managed reimbursement than care. Three common types of managed care organizations are preferred provider organizations (PPOs), group and staff model HMOs, and independent practice association (IPA) HMOs.[2]

**Mean:** The average of a group of numbers.[1]

**Median:** The middle number in a group.[1]

**Medicaid:** A federal-state health insurance program, also enacted in 1965 with Medicare, which covers low-income people who meet variable and changing state eligibility requirements. Most elderly, disabled, and blind individuals who receive assistance through the federal Supplemental Security Income (SSI) program are covered under Medicaid, which is also the main payer of nursing home costs. Federal matching funds to the state range from about 50 to almost 80 percent. Current budget deficits in federal and state budgets threaten this vital safety net program, which provides last-resort coverage for about one in six Americans, including one-fifth of all children in the U.S.[2]

**Medical Home:** This is the term used by all three of our primary care specialties – family medicine, general internal medicine, and general pediatrics – to describe a concept whereby a primary care physician works with a team to provide and coordinate ongoing health care for a patient regardless of the clinical problem. The team forms and reforms according to the needs of the patient, and may include specialists, midlevel providers, nurses, social workers, dieticians, pharmacists, physical and occupational therapists, and others as needed. Continuity of personal and comprehensive health care is assured under this approach.[5]

**Medical Loss Ratio (MLR):** The medical loss ratio is that part of the premium dollar spent on direct medical care. Private insurers typically try to keep their MLR at or below 80%, retaining 20% or more of premium revenue for administrative overhead and profits.[2]

**Medical Necessity:** An elusive but important term which is applied to treatments and health care services which can be judged on the basis of clinical evidence to be effective and indicated as essential medical care. It is an ongoing challenge for health professionals, insurers, payers and policymakers to define medical necessity as part of coverage policy, made more difficult as costs are considered and as new treatments are brought into use.[2]

**Medical Underwriting:** This is the process used by health insurers to calculate higher premiums to be charged to individual or group applicants at higher risk for illness. Medical underwriting was considered unethical in the early years of private insurance in this country, but has become the industry norm, and is usually based on annual review of claims experience.[2]

**Medicare:** A federal insurance program for the elderly and disabled enacted in 1965 which now covers 42 million Americans with benefits including hospital care, physician and other provider services, and limited coverage of the costs of prescription drugs. Medicare beneficiaries include seniors 65 years of age and older, as well as the disabled and those with chronic kidney failure. Traditional (Original) Medicare, as the major source of coverage for one in seven Americans, pays for about one-half of beneficiaries' health care expenses, and accounts for about one-fifth of personal national health expenditures. There are four components of Medicare today:[2]

**Medicare Advantage (MA):** Private health plans authorized by Medicare legislation in 2003 as the sequel to Medicare + Choice programs. Most are HMOs, though recent years have seen an increasing number of preferred provider organizations (PPOs).[2]

Part A    Hospitalization insurance
Part B    Supplementary medical insurance
Part C    Medicare + Choice private plans, now Medicare Advantage
Part D    Prescription drug coverage, starting in 2006

**Medicare + Choice (M + C):** Private health plans authorized by the Balanced Budget Act of 1997 (BBA) intended by their supporters to increase choices available to Medicare beneficiaries. Most were HMOs, with other alternatives including PPOs, provider sponsored organizations (PSOs), and private fee-for-service plans (PFFS).[2]

**Medicare Prescription Drug, Improvement and Modernization Act of 2003 (MMA):** Controversial legislation enacted in 2003 as the most important change in the 40-year life of Medicare. This is a very complex bill, which offers a limited prescription drug benefit while including many other elements which further privatize the program and shift more of its costs from the government to consumers. The pharmaceutical and insurance industries see far more benefits from this bill than Medicare beneficiaries themselves, and future cost projections for Medicare are already surging way beyond initial estimates.[2]

**Medigap:** Private supplementary insurance which covers medical expenses not covered by Medicare, which may include co-payments, deductibles and other related costs. The rising costs of Medigap policies have led to serious underinsurance for many elderly people, with increasing out-of-pocket expenses and difficulties in affording necessary medical care. The annual costs of Medigap policies now run as high as $11,000 per year, and only one in four elderly Americans carry such coverage.[2]

**Mental Health Parity:** Insurance coverage for mental health problems extended on an equal basis with physical, biomedical disorders. The insurance industry has long been wary of such coverage, fearing high demand and adverse selection. It has opposed legislation establishing parity of mental illness, such as the Mental Health Parity Act of 1996 and all later efforts by Congress to extend such legislation.[2]

**Metastasis:** Cancer cells that have spread to one or more sites elsewhere in the body, either regionally to lymph nodes or to distant sites such as the lungs, liver or bones.[1]

**Monopsony Purchasing:** Purchasing of goods and services by a single buyer, such as bulk purchasing of prescription drugs covered by the Veterans

Administration using the leverage of its population to obtain discounted prices from drug manufacturers.[2]

**Moral Hazard:** A concept that gained favor in the 1960s that assumes that people will overuse health care services unless they pay for them directly. Consumers can be made more prudent, the argument goes, by requiring them to pay a portion of these costs out-of-pocket. Based on this concept, together with employers' efforts to trim their exposure to their employees' health care costs, cost-sharing with consumers is increasing. There is abundant evidence, however, which discredits moral hazard as a major cause of health care inflation and recognizes the adverse effects of cost-sharing in restricting access to necessary health care for many lower-income people.[2]

**Mutation:** A change in the DNA of a cell. All types of cancer are thought to be due to mutations that damage a cell's DNA. Most mutations are not passed genetically, but occur after a person is born.[1]

**National Health Insurance (NHI):** A national health insurance program that would provide universal coverage to the entire U.S. population for necessary health care. As with Medicare, NHI would be a single-payer system, government-financed with a private delivery system. Through simplified administration, such a system would provide more efficiency and cost containment than the current market-based system while offering new opportunities to improve accountability and quality assurance within the system.[2]

**Network Providers and Hospitals:** This designation is used by HMOs and PPOs to indicate "preferred providers" within their network of providers and hospitals. What is often marketed by managed care organizations as preferred on the basis of quality is actually preferred on the basis of least costs. Patients are penalized by health plans by paying higher costs if they select out-of-network providers and hospitals.[2]

**Odds Ratio:** This is a measure of the benefit effect of a given intervention; for example, an odds ratio of 1 means that the treatment has no effect; if the odds ratio is less than 1, the treatment has a beneficial effect compared with an intervention applied to a control group; odds ratios of more than 1 mean that the intervention is less effective compared to a control group.[3]

**Outcome:** The consequence of a medical intervention on a patient.[4]

**Overpayment:** Administratively set payments to private Medicare plans in excess of payments to traditional FFS Medicare. These are provided as incentives to bring in and retain more private plans in the Medicare program.

Overpayments belie the notion that private plans save money. Overpayments vary widely around the country, now averaging 112% for Medicare Advantage and ranging up to 132% of FFS Medicare in some high-cost counties.[2]

**Palliative Treatment:** Also called symptom management or comfort care, palliative care is intended to relieve symptoms, such as pain, side effects of treatment, and psychological, social and spiritual problems related to disease; all focused on improving the quality of a patient's life when cure is not expected.[1]

**Part D Prescription Drug Benefit:** Part D is a new component of the Medicare program established in Medicare legislation of 2003 (MMA) whereby partial coverage of prescription drug expenses are provided to Medicare beneficiaries through the private sector.[2]

**Pay-for-Performance (P4P):** P4P initiatives are now in progress among some health plans and as a Medicare demonstration program to test whether reimbursement incentives can result in improved quality of patient care. The jury is still out on the effectiveness of this approach toward quality improvement.[2]

**Point of Service (POS):** Hybrid health plans developed by insurers to give enrollees more choice of providers than provided in conventional HMO plans. Under a POS plan, enrollees are permitted to seek out-of-network care by paying the additional costs out-of-pocket.[2]

**Pre-Existing Condition:** In the process of medical underwriting as insurers evaluate applicants for coverage, medical conditions which pre-date the application are scrutinized as they relate to future health risks. They may be used to deny coverage or to raise initial premiums; if coverage is offered, insurers typically require a six-month waiting period before enrollment.[2]

**Preferred Provider Organization (PPO):** An increasingly popular kind of health plan developed in reaction to many patients' resistance to being locked-in to limited panels of providers. Providers in a PPO panel agree to accept set discounted fees in exchange for the practice-building opportunity of being listed as a "preferred provider."[2]

**Prevalence:** The number of cases of a given disease over a given time period, usually one year.[4]

**Progression-Free Survival:** The length of time a patient has survived without noticeable growth of the cancer.[1]

**Quality-Adjusted Life Year (QALY):** This measure takes into account not only the length of life but also the quality of life during a period of extended life. An analysis using QALYs tries to evaluate the trade-off between mortality, morbidity, and the preference of patients, their families, and society to accept a shortening of life to avoid certain morbidities.[4]

**Randomized Controlled Trials:** These are experimental trials in which people are randomly assigned to an intervention or a control group without an intervention. The randomization refers to allocation among study groups, not to eligibility for the trial.[4]

**Remission:** Complete or partial disappearance of the signs and symptoms of cancer in response to treatment; remission may not be a cure.[1]

**Resource-Based Relative Value Scale (RBRVS):** Under this system, fees for physicians are set for each service by estimating such factors as time, mental effort and judgment, and technical skill involved in each service. RBRVS was adopted by Medicare in the early 1990s in an effort to reduce the wide disparities in reimbursement of procedure-oriented specialists and primary care physicians.[2]

**Risk Pool:** A group of people considered together in order to price their insurance coverage. The larger and more diverse the group in terms of health status, the more effective insurance can be in having healthier individuals share the higher costs of care of sicker individuals while assuring the most affordable insurance premiums for the entire group.[2]

**Severity:** This term describes the stage of disease a patient has.[3]

**Stage:** The extent of a cancer in the body; staging is usually based on the size of the tumor, whether the cancer has spread to the lymph nodes, and whether it has spread from the original site to sites elsewhere in the body.[6]

**State Children's Health Insurance Program (SCHIP):** A federal health insurance program enacted in 1997 as a companion program to Medicaid. SCHIP was initially intended to cover uninsured children in families with incomes at or below 200% of the federal poverty level ($41,300 for a family of four in 2007) but above the traditional income eligibility level for Medicaid. There is wide variation from state to state in these eligibility levels.[2]

**Selective Contracting:** A change during the 1980s when many purchasers and insurers chose to contract selectively with physicians and hospitals, deciding which providers they would pay and which they would not pay. This was intended to hold costs down, and has significantly changed the power relationships among these parties.[2]

**Single-payer:** One health care financing system covering an entire population on the basis of social insurance and replacing a multi-payer system of private insurance. The Medicare program in the U.S. is one such program for the elderly and disabled. Other industrialized countries around the world have their whole populations covered under one or another form of universal health insurance. The U.S. has had such bills put forward in Congress on a number of occasions, including H.R. 676 in the House today, but so far there has not been the political will to overcome the resistance of private stakeholders in our current market-based system.[2]

**Social Insurance:** Social insurance is compulsory, usually provided by a public agency, and spreads the financial risk of illness across an entire population, making its costs affordable to a large population. This is in marked contrast to private insurance, which is voluntary, provided by private insurers (usually for-profit) which selectively enroll better risks, thereby rendering coverage unaffordable or otherwise unavailable to higher-risk individuals. Medicare over the last 40 years has been a social insurance program, but it is threatened by further privatization.[2]

**Targeted Therapy:** Treatment to attack the part of cancer cells that make them different from normal cells. Targeted agents tend to have fewer side effects than conventional chemotherapy drugs.[1]

**Technology Assessment:** This is a form of policy research that evaluates technology in order to provide decision-makers with information on different policy alternatives. These may include the allocation of resources to research and development, development of regulations or legislation, and setting standards or guidelines for health planning and health care practice.[4]

**Underinsurance:** As the costs of health care continue to rise at rates several times the rates of cost-of-living and median family incomes, fewer people can afford insurance with comprehensive benefits. If they can afford coverage at all, they find themselves challenged by high levels of cost-sharing. The Commonwealth Fund has recently defined underinsurance on the basis of the proportion of total family income spent on health care (i.e., more than 10% of income, more than 5% of income if below 200% of federal poverty level, or deductibles equal to or exceeding 5% of income).[2]

**Uninsurance:** This term refers to the growing number, now some 47 million Americans, who have no health insurance, whether private or public. This is a large and heterogeneous group, about one in six of our population. A majority of the uninsured are employed but without affordable coverage or in part-time work without benefits. Many uninsured lose coverage with a recent job change, divorce, or death of a previously insured spouse. Many other uninsured do not qualify for public safety net programs such as Medicaid and SCHIP.[2]

**Universal Coverage:** This term is used to describe countries which provide health insurance to all citizens regardless of age, income, or health status. The U.S. is atypical in not having universal coverage, as illustrated by one in six Americans being uninsured and tens of millions underinsured.[2]

# References:

1. CURE (Cancer Updates, Research & Education), *Cancer Resource Guide*, 2008 Edition. Atlanta, GA, American Cancer Society.
2. Geyman JP. *Do Not Resuscitate: Why the Health Insurance Industry Is Dying, and How We Must Replace It.* Monroe, ME. Common Courage Press, 2008: pp 215-30.
3. Gray JAM. *Evidence-Based Health Care.* New York. Churchill Livingstone, pp 117, 143, 1997.
4. Geyman JP, Deyo RA, Ramsey SD, eds. *Evidence-Based Clinical Practice: Concepts and Approaches.* Boston, MA, 2000, pp 166-72.
5. Rosenthal TC. The medical home: growing evidence to support a new approach to primary care. J *Am Board Fam Med* 21: 427-40, 2008.
6. Hewitt M, Greenfield S, Stovall R, eds. *From Cancer Patient to Cancer Survivor: Lost In Transition.* Washington, DC. The National Academies Press, 2006, pp 477-82.

# APPENDIX 2

# Selected Resources For Cancer Patients

## Information/Education

American Cancer Society...........800-ACS-2345........(800-227-2345)..........www.cancer.org

Cancer Guide ..................................................................................www.cancerguide.org

Cancerfacts.....................................................................................www.cancerfacts.com

Center for Cancer Support & Education .......................................www.centerforcancer.org

CancerCare...................800-813-HOPE....(800-813-4673).................www.cancercare.org

Cancer and Careers................................................................www.cancerandcareers.org

National Cancer Institute ............ 800-4-CANCER ............ (800-422-6237) www.cancer.gov

National Coalition for Cancer Survivorship........877-622-7937......www.canceradvocacy.org

Patient Advocate Foundation.................800-532-5274 ................ www.patientadvocate.org

People Living With Cancer............................703-797-1914............................www.plwc.org

Coalition of National Cancer Cooperative Groups......................www.CancerTrialsHelp.org

Center Watch Clinical Trial Listing Service........................................www.centerwatch.com

## Decision Aids

Foundation for Informed Medical Decision Making ...................................... www.fimdm.org

Healthwise..................................................................................... www.healthwise.org

Mayo Clinic.................................................................................... www.mayoclinic.org

Ottawa Health Research Institute ..................................................www.ohri.ca/decisionaid

## Psychosocial Services

CancerCare............................ 800-813-HOPE ................................. www.cancercare.org

American Psychosocial Oncology Society...........866-276-7443.......www.apos-society.org

The Wellness Community..888-793-WELL/888-793-9355..www.thewellnesscommunity.org

## Palliative Care

The Center to Advance Palliative Care............................................ www.getpalliativecare.org

The National Hospice and Palliative Care Organization................................... www.nhpco.org

## Financial Assistance Programs

Cure Today................................................................................. www.curetoday.com/toolbox
A comprehensive list of financial assistance programs is maintained on this source, including many state governments, drug companies, and other organizations.

# APPENDIX 3

# Frequently Asked Questions About Single-Payer National Health Insurance

**All of these questions and answers are more fully discussed in the text.**

**1. Won't I lose choice with NHI?**

You will have full choice of physicians, other licensed providers, hospitals, and other facilities anywhere in the country under NHI. This will be more choice than you now have with our multi-payer system, which has many ways of limiting choice (e.g. private Medicare plans restricting out-of-network providers).

**2. Won't we have rationing?**

All health care systems ration care in one way or another. Our present system rations care based on ability to pay, excluding many people from essential care. NHI will finance all necessary care for everyone based on medical need, not ability to pay.

**3. Won't NHI cost too much?**

We already have plenty of money in the present system ($2.5 trillion a year and 17.5 percent of GDP). Almost two-thirds of that is already financed by the government. We will save about $380 billion a year by enacting NHI.

**4. Won't quality of care go down with NHI?**

The quality of care for our whole population should improve in a more accountable system with NHI, as universal access without cost-sharing reduces present disparities, encourages prevention, and allows earlier diagnosis and better outcomes of care. Up to one-third of all health care services now being provided in our market-based system are either inappropriate or unnecessary, while millions of Americans go without essential care because of unaffordable costs.

**5. Won't NHI give us more bureaucracy?**

We already have by far the most bureaucratic system in the world, with 1,300 private insurers and many inefficient and diverse plans (e.g., 17,000 different plans in Chicago). NHI will take us to a not-for-profit system with simplified administration and much lower overhead (e.g. overhead of traditional Medicare is 3 percent compared to 19 percent for commercial carriers and 26.5 percent for investor-owned Blues).

**6. Won't NHI stifle innovation?**

Most of the best biomedical research is already carried out by the National Institutes of Health (NIH). That won't change under NHI. Our two single-payer systems that we already have (traditional Medicare and the VA) hardly stifle innovation for their enrollees. Moreover, many advances are made in other countries (e.g. CT scanning in England).

**7. Won't NHI break the bank?**

All other countries with single-payer systems control costs better than we do. Our system is totally out of control with runaway costs, with perverse incentives driving our market-based system to deliver a large amount of services that are inappropriate and unnecessary. Physician-induced demand is a much bigger problem than patients seeking out unnecessary care.

**8. Can we afford NHI?**

Not only can we afford it, but we cannot afford to continue with our present multi-payer system. There is plenty of money in the system. It just needs to be reallocated in a more efficient way, and re-focused on delivering effective and necessary care to everyone who needs it. Enormous ongoing cost savings will be realized by a single-payer financing system through simplified administration, bulk purchasing, use of comparative effectiveness research to inform coverage decisions, and elimination of the wasteful private insurance bureaucracy.

**9. Won't NHI raise my taxes?**

NHI will be funded by a progressive income tax (about 2 percent for most individuals) and an employer payroll tax of about 7 percent. In both cases, this will be less than they are now paying for private coverage through premiums, deductible, co-payments, and the uncovered costs of care. All Americans will get comprehensive coverage for less than they pay now by reallocating the $2.5 trillion already in the system.

**10. Will Americans accept NHI?**

Many opponents of NHI keep telling us that America is unlike most other advanced countries in not needing public financing of health care, that we need a "uniquely American" system consistent with our traditions of individualism and entrepreneurialism. But this myth ignores public opinion surveys that have shown continued majority support for NHI for 50 years, now even including 59 percent of U.S. physicians.

**11. Wouldn't NHI mean a government takeover of health care?**

NHI is a public financing system coupled with a private delivery system. The government pays the bills, but physicians and other health care professionals are in private practice, while most hospitals and other facilities remain in the private sector as they are now. Within a simplified system with less bureaucracy, clinical decisions will be made by patients and their physicians, not the faceless clerks and bureaucrats in today's private insurance.

**12. Isn't NHI socialized medicine?**

NHI is a public financing system coupled with a private delivery system. The government pays the bills, but physicians and other health care

**12. Isn't NHI socialized medicine?** (continued)

professionals are in private practice, while most hospitals and other facilities remain in the private sector as they are now. Within a simplified system with less bureaucracy, clinical decisions will be made by patients and their physicians, not the faceless clerks and bureaucrats in today's private insurance industry. NHI is social insurance, not socialized medicine. England and Spain are examples of socialized medicine, where the government owns and operates hospitals and other facilities and where health professionals are employed by the government. Our traditional Medicare program is publicly financed with private delivery of care, is widely accepted by 45 million Americans enrolled in the program, and is hardly viewed as socialized medicine.

# APPENDIX 4

# Advocacy Organizations For National Health Insurance

## Nurse Organizations

Physicians for a National Health Program: www.pnhp.org

Nurses for single payer: www.guaranteedhealthcare.org,

www.calnurses.org

Everybody (activists) for single payer:

www.healthcare-now.org/

www.pdamerica.org

www..singlepayeraction.org/about.html

Unions for single payer: www.unionsforsinglepayerhr676.org

Leadership Conference for Guaranteed Health Care (national coalition for single payer):

www.guaranteedhealthcare4all.org

## State Organizations

Despite the word "physician in the name of some of these organizations they are open to all. You may wish to connect with the ones closest to you. Here is a list of active organizations, **alphetabetically be state.**

AL     Health Care for Everyone: http://alabamahealthcareforeveryone.org

CA     Nurses Association: www.calnurses.org

**CA     PhysiciansAlliance: http://capa.pnhp.org**

CA     Health Care for All: www.healthcareforall.org

CA     One Care Now: www.onecarenow.org

CO     Health Care for All: www.healthcareforallcolorado.org

DE     Informed Civic/Political Coalition: http://deinformedvoters.org

**CT**        Coalition for Universal Health Care: http://cthealth.server101.com

**DE**        Informed Civic/Political Coalition: http://deinformedvoters.org

**FL**        PNHP: www.tbpnhp.org
**FL**        for Health Security: www.ffhs.org

**GA**        Common Sense Health Plan: www.commonsensehealthplan.org

**IL**         Health Care for All: www.healthcareil.org
**IL**         Single Payer Coalition: www.ilsinglepayercoatition.org

**IN**         Hoosiers for Commonsense Health Plan: www.hchp.info

**KS**        Heartland Health Care forAll: http://healthcareforalLkumc.edu

**KY**        PNHP: www.kyhealthcare.org

**ME**        People's Alliance: www.mainepeoplesalliance.org

**MD**        Health Care for All Coalition: www.mdsinglepayer.org

**MA**        Campaign for Single Payer. www.masscare.org
**MA**        Affordable Health Insurance for Everyone: http://healthcareformass.org
**MA**        Alliance to Defend Health Care: www.massdefendhealthcare.org

**MI**         Universal Health Care Access Network: www.michuhcan.com

**MN**        Universal Health Care Coalition: www.muhcc.org
**MN**        Citizens Organized Acting Together: www.coact.org
**MO**        for Single Payer Healthcare: www.mosp.us

**MS**        PNHP: www.pnhp-mo.org

**NH**      PNHP: http://nh.pnhp.org

**NY**      Metro Chapter of PNHP: pnhpnymetro.org

**NY**      State Capital District PNHP: http://capitaldistrictpnhp.blogspot.com

**NC**      Committee to Defend Health Care: www.ncdefendhealthcare.org

**NC**      Health Care for A11 North Carolina: www.HealthCareforAllNC.org

**OH**      Single Payer Action Network: www.spanohio.org

**OH**      PNHP Ohio www.pnhpohio.org

**OH**      Health Care for All Ohio: http://healthcareforallohio.org

**OR**      Health Care for All: www.healthcareforalloregon.org

**PA**      Philly Area Committee to Defend Health Care: www.phillyhealth.org

**PA**      http://phillyhealth.blogspot.com

**RI**      Everybody In Nobody Out: www.everybodyinnobodyout.org

**TX**      Health Care for All: www.healthcareforalltexas.org

**UT**      Health Alliance: www.utahhealthalliance.org

**VT**      Health Care for All: www.vthca.org

WA      Health Care for All: www.healthcareforallwa.org

**WA**      PNHP: www.pnhpwesternwashington.org

**WV**      Mountain State PNHP: http://mountainstatepnhp.com

**WI**      Coalition for Health: www.wisconsinhealth.org

**WY**      Voices Foundation: www.wyoming-voices.org

**More State Contacts:**

Healthcare Now.............................................www.healthcare-now.org

# Index

AARP position on reform, 247
Adler, Nancy, 88
Aetna, 199(Table 10.2),200(Fig. 10.2)
affordability. *See* costs
African-Americans, cancer rates and
    deaths, 35, 83, 84, 85, 124
Agency for Healthcare Policy and
    Research (AHCPR), 129
Agency for Healthcare Research and
    Quality (AHRQ), 76, 129, 174, 211,
    263
aging
    cancer and, 82
    and co-morbidity, 127-128
    guidelines for screening, 128
    (Table 7.1)
    Medicare role, 167
Alaska Natives, survival rates, 84
Albertson, Dr. Peter, 45
Alliance Packaging, 186-187
Allstate cancer policy, 109, 168
Altman, Drew, 108
American Board of Medical
    Specialties, 89
American Cancer Society (ACS)
    cancer projections, 17
    costs, prohibitive, study, 174
    "4-As" program, 18, 35, 127, 165–
    166, 189, 221, 231, 246
    Health Insurance Assistance
    Service, 18
    MRI recommendations, 45
    national call center, 166-167
    National Data Base, 101–102, 103,
    107–108
    public relations campaign for
    screening, 18
    screening study, 101-102
    smoking statistics, 86, 145-146
    *Spending to Survive* cases, 30
    survivor concerns, 87 (Fig. 4.1) –88

American College of Emergency
    Physicians (ACEP), 217
American College of Physicians, 241
American College of Radiology
    (ACR), 46, 125, 153
American Hospital Association costs,
    71
American Human Development
    Project, 232
American Indians, survival rates, 84
American Medical Association study of
    HMO/PPO insurance, 142, 201
America's Health Insurance Plans
    (AHIP), 172, 199, 263
American Society of Clinical Oncology
    (ASCO), 26, 82, 94
American Society for Therapeutic
    Radiology and Oncology, 150
American Human Development Report,
    231, 232
Amgen, 49, 154
Angell, Dr. Marcia, 172
Anthem Blue Cross plan, example, 109
Aranesp, 50, 126, 154
Arrow, Kenneth, 141
Ascension Health, 147
association health plans (AHPs),
    172, 209, 263
Avastin, 48, 53, 54, 93, 94, 109, 126,
    128, 131, 152

baby boomers, 261–262
    cancer in, 17
    geriatrics shortage for, 241
    risks in, 17
Bach, Dr. Peter, 126
bait and switch, 149, 209
Baker, Dean, 236, 237
bankruptcy filings by seniors, 63
Bartlett, Mike, 198
Baucus, Senator Max, 235, 249, 252,
    253 (Figure 11.1)

Bennett, Dr. Charles, 50
bevacuzumab. *See* Avastin
Big 5 health insurance industry players,
    199 (Table 10.2), 200 (Figure 10.2)
bioethics in cancer care, 242–244
biomedical research / industry,
    214, 236
bladder cancer, 34
Blue Cross
    bank, 198
    "catastrophic" plan, 109
    as Medicare intermediary, 151, 240
Blue Cross of California, 70
Blue Cross Blue Shield Association
    (Chicago), 213
Blue Cross-Blue Shield of Michigan,
    94
Blue Cross Blue Shield Technology
    Evaluation Committee, 214
Boylan, Dr. Laura, 233
Bradley, U.S. Senator Bill, 193, 194
Braly, Angela, 143
BRCA 1 and BRCA 2 genes,
    43–45, 47-48
breast cancer
    African-Americans with, 85, 103
    *Archives of Internal Medicine* study
        on, 119
    British comparison to U.S., 114,
        116
    decisions, 92 (Table 4.1)
    diagnosis, international comparison,
        114
    drugs, 43 (Table 2.1)
    by ethnicity, 84
    incidence, 27
    mammogram study, 119
    radiation for, 245
    risks, 44
    screening, 45, 117
    treatment, 48, 93
Bristol-Myers Squibb, 214
Brook, Robert, 126
Budetti, Dr. Peter, 158
Bureau of Labor

estimates of 65 and older, 65–66
    report on COBRA premiums, 76
Bush Administration regulation of
    cancer therapies, 49

CA-125 blood tests, 44–45
California Department of Managed
    Health Care, 70
Callahan, Daniel, 140
Canada, health care, 85, 187, 201
    compared to U.S., 113, 116, 183
        (Fig. 9.2), 202–203
    costs, 182, 216
    wait times, 217–219 (Fig. 10.4)
Canada's Common Drug Review, 235
cancer. *See also* costs; diagnosis;
                drugs; prevention; screening;
                therapy; rationing; risks;
                treatment; specific cancers.
    baby boomers with, 239
    care in U.S., 34, 35, 81, 82–83, 86,
        94, 113, 118
    cost-effective, 129
    disparities in, 124–125
    ethical issues in, 242–244
    in free market, 158–159
    one-tier, 231, 233
    centers, 27, 239
    in children, 32, 35
    cross-national comparisons,
        113–115
    cures, 18, 39
    death rates / mortality,
        27, 29, 32, 33–34, 36, 86
    decision-making, shared, 90–92
    fast-growing and slow-growing, 117
    gender incidence, men and women,
        28, 34, 82
    hereditary, 44
    historical landmarks / benchmarks,
        25–27
    minority beliefs about, 85
    in older people, 82, 127, 167, 236
    OOPE for, 173–174
    origin of term, 26
    policy, 52–53, 55–56, 129–31

prevalence by age group,
28 (Fig. 1.1)–29
as projected #1 chronic disease and
leading cause of death,
5, 30, 82, 227
registries, 94
research and research aims,
155–158, 233, 236, 244
resources, 277 (Appendix 2)
risks, 82, 228
socioeconomic status, and cancer,
35
survivors, 32, 33 (Fig. 1.3), 34, 35,
36, 48, 114, 117, 118, 119
care, 103
concerns, 87 (Fig. 4.1)–88
insurance of, 67, 102 (Fig. 5.2)
lead-time bias, 116-118
leukemia, 114
number of, 87
primary care for, 241–242
and quality of life, 129
Cancer Cooperative Group, 238
Cancer Genome Anatomy Project
(CGAP), 27
Cancer Trends Progress Report (NCI),
34–35
Caplan, Arthur, 55
carcinoma, origin and meaning of term,
24
CareCredit debt, 73
Carilion Health System, 152
CBO (Congressional Budget Office)
reports, 62, 148, 186 (Table 9.3),
196, 208, 209, 219–220, 234, 252,
253
Center on Budget & Policy Priorities,
173
Center for Economic and Policy
Research, 236
Center for Responsive Politics, 249
Center for Studying Health System
Change, 63
Centers for Disease Control and
Prevention

ER visits, report, 217
NPCR-CSS, 94
2008 Annual Report to the Nation,
34–36
certification
in medical oncology, 26–27
in radiation oncology, 27
cetuximab. *See* Erbitux
Champaign County Health Care
Consumers, 73
ChaseHealthAdvance, 73
chemotherapy
anti-anemia drugs in, 49, 53, 55, 71,
74, 126, 154, 244
clinical trials, 92
counseling in late stages, 244
cytotoxic / traditional, 48
costs, example, 125
drugs
costs of, 20, 124, 133
excluded, 74
rebated, 55, 154, 244
genetic information in, 46
Medicaid involvement, 173
side-effects, 94
chronic disease management, 208–209
Cigna, 200 (Fig. 10.2)
Claxton, Gary, 74
Clinical Effectiveness Program,
proposed, 233, 234
*Clinical Epidemiology* (Sackett,
Haynes, Guyatt, Tugwell), 116
clinical practice guidelines (CPGs),
238–239
clinical trials, 92–93, 94, 174–175, 214,
236, 237–238
example, 175
CMS (Center for Medicare and
Medicaid Services, 264
estimates of medical care, 73
for Medicare, 239
research, 237
Coalition of Cancer Cooperative
Groups, 238
Coast Institutional Review Board

(Colorado), 244
COBRA insurance, 32, 75-76, 251, 264
colon / colorectal cancers, 18, 29, 44,
    46, 48, 85, 90, 91, 94, 126, 179, 204
colonoscopy, 46, 90, 152
Comis, Dr. Robert, 238
Common Drug Review (Canada),
    130, 235
Commonwealth Fund reports, 60, 112,
    201, 202, 203(Fig. 10.3), 215, 216
community health centers, 241, 264
Community Tracking Study (CTS), 144
co-morbidities, 33, 82, 83, 87, 103-104,
    127, 264
    in older adults, 127–128
Comparative Effectiveness Institute,
    235, 237, 239, 240
conflicts of interest (COIs), 156, 236,
    238, 242, 244, 245, 248
Conrad, Senator, Kent 235
Conrad Hilton Foundation, 231
Conservatives for Patients' Rights, 250
consolidation / competition in
    marketplace, 141–142,
        143 (Fig. 8.1), 145
consumer confidence, 65
consumer-directed health care (CDHC),
    205–206, 264
contagion, early fears of, 26
Conyers, Rep. John, Jr., 250
co-payments, 71, 107-109, 265
    example, 70–71
cost, cancer / health, 66, 168, 174.
    *See also* insurance
    Canada comparison, 113, 118,
        183 (Fig. 9.2), 202–203
    of CT scanning, 40–41
    of drugs, 66, 93, 114, 123, 131, 168
    Medicare, 167–168
    NIH projected, 216
    per-capita, in U.S., 185 (Fig. 9.4)
    projected, 30
    rising, 17, 19, 20, 54, 55, 81, 83,
        122, 123, 129, 169, 248
      screening, 46

single-payer, 182–183, 216
    of targeted therapies, 48
    of technology, 41, 52
    trends, 81
cost-containment, 121, 179, 208, 210,
    216
cost-effectiveness, 235, 244
cost-sharing, 178, 207, 209, 215, 265
Courtney, Michael, case, 31–32
coverage with evidence development
(CED), 235
CT (computerized tomography)
    scanning, 46–47, 153, 154
    costs, 234, 240
    of smokers, 157
Cullen, Kevin J., 81
cures, cancer, 18, 39

darbepbepoetin alpha. *See* Aranesp
Dartmouth Institute for Health Policy
    and Clinical Practice, 119
Dartmouth Medical School Study, 204
Datamonitor, international comparison,
    114
Dave case (insurance denied), 105-106
Davis, Neil, 19
decision-making, shared,
    90–92 (Table 4.1), 242–243
Department of Health and Human
    Services (DHHS), 27, 155-156
Desmond-Hellmann, Dr. Susan, 152
diagnosis, 82, 83, 113, 116, 178
    of breast cancer, 43, 47
    early, 34, 115, 117
    false-positive, 42
    late, and survival, 103–104
        (Fig. 5.2)
    rates, 33
disease management(DM),
    208, 265–266
*Do Not Resuscitate* (Geyman),
    20, 168–169, 171,
        180 (Table 9.2), 185
"doughnut hole," 149
Drazen, Dr. Jeffrey, 157

Drexel University's Clinical Trials
   Research Center, 238
drugs, cancer, 34, 42, 43, 122–123,
155, 214. *See also* chemotherapy
   anti-anemia, 48–49, 55, 126, 154–
      155, 244
   companies, 238
   costs, 93, 114, 123, 131, 168, 201
   and benefits of, 41 (Table 2.1)
   "doughnut hole," 149
   guidelines for, 239
   for lung cancer, 158
   off-label, 49
   Medicaid, 251
   for oral cancer, 149
   prescription, 64, 71, 178
   research, 93
   targeted, 48-49, 53

Einstein, Albert, 165
electronic medical records (EMRs),
   207–208
Elmendorf, Douglas, 253
emergency room services / visits,
   101, 105, 147, 179, 215, 217, 248
employer-sponsored coverage,
   108, 170 (Fig. 9.1), 176
England
   comparison with U.S., 54, 204, 213
   as CT scanning developer, 213
Epoetin alpha. *See* Procrit
Epogen, 50
Erbitux, 123, 126
Erlotinib, 114
Erwin, Deborah, 86
ESAs, 49–50
esophagus cancer, 34, 35
ethical issues, 233, 242–244
ethnicity. *See* minorities
Euripides, 262
EUROCARE data.
   *See* Lancet Oncology
Evans, Dr. James, 56–57
Evans, Robert, 141, 178, 206, 210–211
*Evidence-Based Health Care* (Muir

Gray), 116

Fairness & Accuracy in Reporting
   (FAIR), 250
Families USA report, 209
family medicine, 83
Federal Drug Administration (FDA),
   42, 56
   approvals, 45, 46, 50, 128–129,
      156, 157
   politics and restrictions, 234, 244,
      245
   regulation of tobacco, 86
   research, 237
Federal Employees Health Benefits
   Program (FEHBP), 68
fee-for-service (FFS), 240, 267
Fein, Dr. Oliver, 250
Ferrell, Betty, 89
Fisher, Dr. Elliott, 41 (Fig. 2.1),
   153–154
for-profit health care system,
   failures of, 17, 241, 244
Fox Chase Cancer Center, 49
Fraser Institute, 217–218
free market, 139–140, 159–160, 193,
   195 (Table 10.1), 196–198, 229,
   239, 250
   accountability, 205
   and cancer patients, 141
   lobbying for, 248–249–250
   monopolies, 201–202
   opposition to single-payer, 211–212
   regulation of, 244
   reimbursement policies, 238
GAO report, 196
gastric cancers, 44
Genentech, 152–153
genetic testing / medicine, 40–44, 54
geriatrics
   oncology, 233, 241
   shortage, 241
   specialty, 83, 240
Gingrich, Newt, 139–140
Gleevec, 39, 48

Goethe, 228
Goodman, Dr. Steven, 237
Gould, Stephen Jay, 243
graduate medical education (GME), 242
Gray, Dr. J. A. Muir, 116
Group Health Cooperative, 208
Gruber, Jonathan, 196
Guardasil, 69
Guyatt, Gordon, 116

Harvard University
    costs study, 65
    insurance study, 67
    School of Public Health study, 107, 106 (Fig. 5.3)
Hayek, Dr. Friedrich A., 227, 228
Haynes, Brian, 116
HCA, Inc., 250
health care, 113, 159–160, 253.
    *See also* costs, cancer; reform
    ACA's goal, 246
    access to, 61–62, 102 (Table 5.1), 165, 166
    accountability, 244
    best countries for, 202, 203
    costs by household income share, 186
    debate, reframing, 228–230
    financing, 110
    lobbying, 248
    mandates, 206–207
    myths, 194, 195 (Table 10.1), 238
    rising costs of, 61, 83, 248
Health Care Summit (2009), 250
health insurance. *See* insurance
Health Net, 70
health savings accounts (HSAs), 198, 268
Healthy New York insurance plan, 31
heart disease
    death rates from, 27
    as number one killer, 17
Held, Mark, 187
Henschke, Dr. Claudia, 156-157

Herceptin, 43–44, 48, 109, 110
HER2 gene, 43–44, 128
high-risk pools, 209
Himmelstein, Dr. David, 144–145, 210
HIPPA rules governing pre-existing condition exclusions, 31–32
Hippocrates, description of cancer, 26
Hispanic/Latino
    cancer care, 85
    uninsured, 67, 124
HMOs (Health Maintenance Organizations), 144 (Table 8.1), 179, 196, 204, 208, 268
Hodgkin's disease, 31, 35, 39
hospital(s)
    admission example, 72–73
    HCA as for-profit chain, 249–250
    mortality in hospital, 107–108
    Nevada public, 84-85
    not-for-profit, 72, 147–148, 204
human development index (HDI), 231–232
human experimentation companies (HECs), 244
Humana
    drug plan, 149
    reimbursement cuts, 198
    share values, 199 (Table 10.2), 200 (Fig. 10.2)

Iacocca, Lee, 186
imaging centers / services / procedures, 46, 153–154, 234, 244
imatinib, 39
IMS Health, 64
income, average, 64 (Fig. 3.2)
information technology (IT), 207–208
Institute of Medicine
    cancer projections, 29
    geriatrician shortage, documentation, 241
    insurance report, 68
    quality of care definition, 126
    uninsured, 67
insurance. *See also* multi-payer;

national health insurance; private insurance
and health care access, 100 (Table 5.1)
benefits, limited, 109
caps/limits, 74, 168
cash and carry, 71–72
costs, 68
coverage, 110
denied, 68–69, 168
deductibles, 168, 265
employer-based, 233
examples, 19, 20, 67, 68–69, 70, 74–75, 107
inadequate, 18, 20, 63, 65, 66
premiums, 69 (Fig. 3.3), 108, 142, 149, 168, 169, 173
unavailable or losing, 68, 176
investor-owned care, 144 (Table 8.1)

Jefferson, Thomas, 39, 262
Johnson & Johnson, 77, 154
Joint Commission on the Accreditation of Healthcare Orgnizations (JCAHO), 245

Kaiser Commission on Medicaid and the Uninsured, 215–216
Kaiser Family Foundation, 18
costs surveys, 65, 108–109
coverage/caps, 74
households affected by cancer study, 105
insurance study, 67
Taylor Wilhite and Michael Courtney cases, 30–32
Kaiser Permanente, 208
Karlin case (insurance cap), 74–75
Kassirer, Dr. Jerome, 157
Kennedy, Dr. B.J, 82
Kennedy, John F., 194
Kessler, Dr. David, 237
kidney cancer, 35, 66
King, Dr. Martin Luther, 255
Knome, 145

Krugman, Paul, 189, 212, 221

Laboratory Corporation of America, 43
Lakoff, George, 229
*Lancet Oncology* cross-national reports, 34, 35, 36, 113, 114, 115
Leadership Conference for Guaranteed Health Care, 254
lead time, or length bias, 116, 117
Lennhoff, Claudia, 73
leukemia, 35
example, 39
treatment, 39, 48
Lewis, Kristen, 232
life expectancy, 232
Lincoln, Abraham, 193, 194
Lindert, Peter, 153
liver cancer, 34, 35
*The Lives of the Cell: Notes of a Biology Watcher* (Thomas), 40
longevity, 243
lung cancer, 29, 48, 85, 146, 157, 158
lymphoma, 48

Machiavelli, Niccolo di Bernardo, 165
Malthusian view, 61
mammography / mammograms, 44, 46, 102, 114, 120
MammoSite, 245
market / marketplace. *See* free markets
Massachusetts Medical Society, 217
"Massachusetts Miracle" mandate, 201–207
Matloff, Ellen, 46
McCanne, Dr. Don, 230
McCaughey, Betsy, 34
McDonalds, insurance, 200–201
McGlynn, Elizabeth, 126
McLesky, Sandra, 127
M. D. Anderson Cancer Center, 72–73
*Measure of America*, 231
*The Median Isn't the Message* (Gould), 243
Medicaid, 76, 10, 169, 172–173, 254,

269
cost-sharing, 107, 173
coverage of poor, 84–85
cuts, 248
diagnosis, late, 103
drugs, 251
in Missouri, 173
in Utah, 173
overhead, 173
stimulus package spending for, 251
Medical Association of the State of
New York, 213
medical bankruptcy, 174. *See also* costs
medical care costs, 61, 63, 65, 73, 77.
*See also* costs, cancer
Medical Expenditure Panel surveys,
174
medical-loss ratios (MCRs), 143, 270
medical technologies, 39, 57
benefits versus harms, 42
harms of, 41 (Fig. 2.1)
levels (Thomas), 40
melanoma, 44
Medicare, 130, 151–152, 158, 167–
168, 169, 213, 245, 254, 270
access to, 101
Blue Cross as intermediary for, 152,
240
cost-effectiveness, 235
coverage, 49, 66
drug spending, 122, 126, 251
laws governing, 234
numbers in, 235
overhead, 213
Part D, 237, 270, 272
plans, 148–150
private, 196, 198, 212, 252
wait times, 219
Medicare Advantage, 74, 148, 149,
199, 271–272
Medicare for All, 77, 110, 233, 252
Medicare Payment Advisory
Commission (MedPAC), 149, 150,
234
Medicare Prescription Drug,

Improvement, and Modernization
Act of 2003 (MMA), 148, 271
Medicare Rights Center, Private Health
Plan Monitoring Project, 178
Medigap, 109, 271
mental health centers, 144 (Table 8.1)
Meropol, Dr. Neal, 123
Meyskens, Frank L., Jr., 81
"Millennials," 254.
*See also* baby boomers
Milliman Medical Index, 210
minorities
cancer care among, 84, 85, 227
late diagnosis in, 124
*Mired in the Health Care Morass*
(Davis), 19–20
monoclonal antibodies, 48
mortality
comparison by country,
202–203 (Fig. 10.3)
from drugs, 50
by ethnicity and gender, 83–84
in-hospital, 107–108
MRI screening, 44, 47, 234
multi-payer
financing, 166–167, 175–176, 179,
187 (Table 9.4), 189, 195
(Table 10.1), 199–202, 229, 230
reform, 205, 248 (Table 11.2)
myeloma, 35, 48

Nanospectra Biosciences, 52
nanotechnology, 42, 51–52
National Association for Proton
Therapy (NAPT), 150
National Cancer Act of 1971, 26, 27
National Cancer Data Base (NCDB),
101–102
National Cancer Institute (NCI), 26,
34, 81, 92, 118
Cancer Trends Progress Report
(2008), 33–35
Center to Reduce Cancer Health
Disparities, 35
clinical trials, 238

mission of, 27
randomized trials position, 118
research, 30, 251
2008 Annual Report to the Nation, 33
National Cancer Program, 25
National Center for Policy Analysis (NCPA)
cancer rate study, 34
on free markets, 193
on rationing, 216
on wait times, 218
National Comprehensive Cancer Network (NCCN), 239
National Federation of Independent Business, 142
national health insurance (NHI), 177–178, 179–186, 272. *See also* single-payer system
advocacy organizations, 283 (Appendix 4)
bureaucracy, 212–213
costs, 220
paradigm shift for, 245
questions frequently asked, 279 282
rationing, 219
support for, 253
universal coverage through, 231
winners and losers, 186–189
National Institutes of Health, 156, 214, 237
National Institute for Health and Clinical Excellence (NICE), 54, 130, 235
National Roundtable on Health Care Quality, 126
National Survey of Households Affected by Cancer, 105
Navigenics, 145
Nevpogen, 71
Newcomer, Dr. Lee, 19, 48–49, 57
Non-Hodgkin lymphoma (Michael Courtney case), 31, 35, 115
nonprofit organizations devoted to

cancer, 30
Noonday Global Management, 53
North American Association of Central Cancer Registries, 33–34
not-for-profit
ACS position on, 246
Blue Cross Blue Shield of Michigan, 198
care, 144 (Table 8.1), 151, 210
HMOs, 208
hospitals, 72, 147–148, 204
NCCN as, 239
public financing, 232
Novello, Dr. Antonia, 84
nursing home care, 144 (Table 8.1)
Nyman, John, 215

Obama (President) public plan, 250, 251
Office of National Health Information Technology Coordinator, 207
oncology/oncologists
concerns, 54–55, 81, 82–83, 90, 130–131
drugs, 122
education, 82
geriatric, 233
gynecologic, 26–27
Goodman, Dr. Steven, 237
and Medicare reimbursement, 173
for older people, 239
rebates, drug, 154
on Tumor Boards, 242
oral cancer drugs, 149
Orszag, Peter, 234, 235
out-of-pocket (OOP) expenditures, 73–74, 173–174, 177, 196
ovarian cancer, 44–45
OvaSure, 45
Ovation Pharmaceuticals, 66
overpayments, 197, 212, 272
Oxfam America, 231

Pacific Research Institute, 53
palliative care, 86, 88–89, 178, 243

pancreatic cancer, 48, 93, 204
Pap smears, percentage getting, 114
Part D. *See* Medicare
Partnership to Improve Patient Care,
    249
patient assistance program, 175
patient education, 208
Patrick, Governor Deval, 207
pay, ability to, 63, 64
payroll tax, 184
PET imaging, 66, 153, 234
Pew Research Center, 220–221
Philip Morris International, 146
photothermal ablation, 52
physicians, access to,
    99–100 (Fig. 5.1), 101
Physicians for a National Health
    Program (PNHP), 230, 250
Pipes, Sally, 53–54
poverty, and cancer care, 85, 86, 87
pre-existing conditions, 273
    coverage for, 176
    example, 31–32
    HIPAA rules governing, 31
prescription drugs. *See* drugs
prevention, cancer, 27, 40, 55, 82, 86,
    131, 182, 233, 236, 239, 251
primary care
    and oncology coordination, 89–90
    for cancer survivors, 241–242
    in Massachusetts, 217
    NIH and, 182
    proposals for, 233, 239
    shortage, 101, 241
private insurance, 138, 139, 168, 169,
    170 (Table 9.1), 171–172, 177, 179,
    190, 198, 199–200, 209, 211, 213,
    227, 233. *See also* free market
    and delivery system, 246
    clinical trials, 236
    defenders, 250
    inefficiencies of, 228, 248
    20/80 rule, 197
Procrit, 50, 71, 126, 154
ProCure Treatment Centers, 51, 150

profit motives, 193.
    *See also* free market
progression-free survival (PFS), 237
prostate cancer, 43, 115
    costs, 20
    drugs, 56
    genetic testing for, 44
    incidence, 20, 29
    orchiectomy for, 91
    proton therapy for, 51, 151
    risks, 45
    screening for, 45
    survival rates, 115–116
prostatectomy, 125–126, 127
proton
    accelerators, 20, 50
    therapy, 50–51, 150–151
Provenge, 56
psychiatry specialty, 240
Public Citizen's Health Research
    Group, 76, 85, 177
public financing, 183–184, 236, 246
public health insurance, 177.
    *See also* national health insurance
Public Health Service, 27
public plan option vs single-payer,
    253 (Fig. 11.2)

QALY (quality-adjusted life years), 52,
    54, 55, 56, 129, 130, 131, 265, 273
quality of care, 125, 126–127, 129, 179
    budget to improve, 251
    comparison among countries, 204–
        205, 208
    in free market, 239
quality control, laboratory, 44

radiation. *See also* proton therapy
    for breast cancer, 245
    by ethnic group, 85
    exposure, 47, 125
    with older women, 101
    study by ACS, 101
    therapists on boards, 242
    therapy, 50

raloxifene, 86, 94
RAND reports
    disease management, 208
    on cost-sharing, 215
    on health care spending, 123
Ramsey, Dr. Scott, 130
randomized trials, 117
rationing, 131–132, 195 (Table 10.1), 210–211, 249, 279
Rawlins, Sir Michael, 54
reform, health care, 21, 193, 205, 207, 210, 228–230, 240, 245, 248, 250, 251, 252, 254
    activism, 261–262
reimbursement policies and reform, 239–230, 240, 242, 246
Reinhardt, Uwe, 220
Relman, Dr. Arnold, 241
Resnick, Barbara, 127
risks, cancer
    aging as, 17
    ESAs as, 50
    genetic screening for, 44–45
*The Road to Serfdom* (Hayek), 227
R J Reynolds, 146
Robert case (AARP plan), 107
Roberts, Dr. Thomas, 53
Robinson, James, 71
robotic surgery, 42
Rockefeller Foundation, 231
Rockridge Institute Report, 229
Ross, Lainie Friedman, 99
Roosevelt, Franklin D., 26
Roswell Park Cancer Institute, 86
Ryan, Rep. Paul, 139

Sackett, Dr. David, 116, 117
safety net, 75–76
SCHIP (State Children's Health Insurance Program), 212, 250, 274
Schulman, Kevin, 123
Scott, Richard, 249
Schuster, Mark, 126
screening, 36, 82, 86, 101–102, 114, 178
    for colon cancer, 92
    CT scans, 46, 125
    funding for, 236
    genetic testing in, 42–46
    and insurance status, 102– (Table 5.2)103
    international comparison, 113, 114
    in older adults, 127, 128 (Table 7.1), 239
    for prostate cancer, 125
*A Second Opinion* (Relman), 241
Seffrin, John, 166
self-employment example, 67–68
self-pay, 173–174
self-referral, 240, 244
Sen, Amartya, 231
Siminoff, Laura A., 99
Simone, Joseph V., 121, 122
Sinclair, Upton, 151
single-payer system, 77, 178, 180 (Table 9.2), 182, 187 (Table 9.4), 189, 228–230, 252, 253. *See also* national health insurance
    advocates for reform, 250
    costs, 216
    administrative, 252–253 (Figure 11.2)
    CPGs under, 239
    definition, 274
    financing, 176, 178
    for future, 247 (Table 11.2)
    Medicare for All, 233
    opponents, 210, 213, 248, 250
    reimbursement reform in, 240
    suggested requirements, 229–230
Sinibaldi, John, 171
small molecular inhibitors, 48
smoking and cessation, 86, 146
    and CT scan of lungs, 157
socialized medicine, 211–212, 250, 282–282
Society of Gynecologic Oncologists, 45
Sophocles, 127
Southern California Kaiser Permanente Oncology Research Program, 94

*Spending to Survive* (NCI), 18, 30
spontaneous remission, 119
Sprycel, 107
Starfield, 205
Stiglitz, Dr. Joseph, 159
Sulmasy, Dr. Daniel, 127, 132
Sweden R & D, 214

Taiwan, insurance coverage,
    184 (Fig. 9.3)
Taplin, Dr. Stephen, 118
taxes for health care, 219,
    220 (Fig. 10.5)
Taxol, 54, 214
technology. *See* medical technologies
Tenet, 72, 142
testicular cancer, 39
therapy
    anti-anemia, 49–50
    individualized, 52
    proton, 50–51
    radiation, 50
    targeted, 48–49, 50
Thomas, Lewis, 40
Thomson Reuters, 124
thyroid, 35
tobacco, 103, 165. *See also* smoking
    industry, 143–144
Tom's case (leukemia), 39
transvaginal ultrasounds, 44
trastuzumab, 43
treatment, cancer, 27, 46, 55, 86, 114,
    167
    for baby boomers and older people,
    239
    overemphasis on, 86–87
    radiation, 48, 93, 245
    refusing, for cost reasons, 124
    shared decision-making in, 91
    versus prevention, 86
TrialCheck, 238
Tugwell, Peter, 116
Tumor Boards, 242
Tumulty, Karen, 248
23andMe, 145

20/80 rule, 197 (Fig. 10.1)
Tykerb, 71, 109

Ullrich, Dr. Christopher, 153
ultrasound screening, 47
unemployment benefits, lack of, 65
uninsured and underinsured, 61, 62
    (Fig. 3.1), 65, 84, 99, 106–107, 206,
    211, 248, 275
    and diagnosis, late, 126
    in Los Angeles County, 217
    OOPE for cancer care, 174–175
    in private insurance, 170 (Table 9.1)
    screening, lack of, 103
    survivor care, 105
United Health
    AARP association, 248
    anti-anemia drug study, 126
    banks, 198
    stock values (Fig. 10.2)
United Healthcare
    caps, 74
    and genetic testing, 44
    and targeted therapies, 48–49
United States National Health
    Insurance (USNHI), 178
United Nations' Universal Declaration
    of Human Rights, 229
universal health care coverage, 172,
    179, 184, 207, 210, 231, 275.
    *See also* national health insurance
University Medical Center, Las Vegas,
    Nevada, 36
*USA Today* cancer study, 105
U.S. National Health Care Act, 250

Veterans Administration (VA), 148,
    158, 181, 212, 213, 237
"volunteer effect," 116–117
von Goethe, Johann Wolfgang, 227

Wagoner, G. Richard, Jr., 186
wait times, 217, 218 (Fig. 10.4)
    in Canada, 219
Wal-mart insurance, 200–201

*Washington Post* costs survey, 65
Wasunna, Angela, 140
Weissman, Robert, 146
Welch, Dr. Gilbert, 41 (Fig. 2.1)
WellCare, 74
Wellpoint, 70, 200 (Fig. 10.2)
Wender, Dr. Richard, 165, 166–167
Wharam, Dr. Frank, 127
White, Dr. Kerr, 30
Wilbur, Ray Lyman, 121, 122, 131
Williams, Dr. Timothy, 150
Wilms' tumor, 66
Wolfe, Dr. Sidney, 177
Woolhandler, Steffie, 144–145
World Health Organization reports
    on leukemia survival rates, 114
    on prevention of deaths, 84
WSHIP example, 109

x-ray therapy, 50

Yale Cancer Center, 46, 85–86

Zeitman, Dr. Anthony, 51
zero-time shift, 117

# About the Author

John Geyman, M.D. is Professor Emeritus of Family Medicine at the University of Washington School of Medicine in Seattle, where he served as Chairman of the Department of Family Medicine from 1976 to 1990. As a family physician with over 25 years in academic medicine, he has also practiced in rural communities for 13 years. He was the founding editor of *The Journal of Family Practice* (1973 to 1990) and the editor of *The Journal of the American Board of Family Practice* from 1990 to 2003. His most recent books are *Health Care in America: Can Our Ailing System Be Healed?* (Butterworth-Heinemann, 2002), *The Corporate Transformation of Health Care: Can the Public Interest Still Be Served?* (Springer Publishing Company, 2004), *Falling Through the Safety Net: Americans Without Health Insurance* (2005), *Shredding the Social Contract: The Privatization of Medicare* (2006), *The Corrosion of Medicine: Can the Profession Reclaim its Moral Legacy?* (2008), *Do Not Resuscitate: Why the Health Insurance Industry is Dying, and How We Must Replace It* (2008), *Hijacked: The Road to Single Payer in the Aftermath of Stolen Health Care Reform (*2010), and *Breaking Point: How the Primary Care Crisis Endangers the Lives of Americans* (2011). Dr. Geyman served as President of Physicians for a National Health Program from 2005 to 2007 and is a member of the Institute of Medicine.

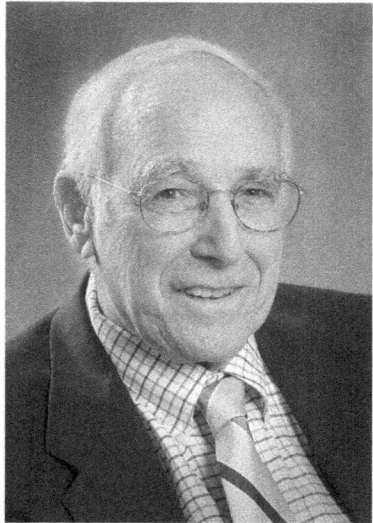

# *Understanding the Big Picture:*

Taken together, *The Cancer Generation* and six other volumes by John Geyman from Copernicus Health Care show in vivid detail how health care has become just another commodity in our market-based non-system, and how soaring costs exclude many millions of Americans from necessary care. These books also offer concrete directions for reforms which can control costs and provide access to health care that all Americans can depend upon.

**Falling Through the Safety Net: Americans Without Health Insurance**
2005 / 224 pages, $18.95, ISBN 1??

**Shredding the Social Contract: The Privatization of Medicare**
2006 / 322 pages, $16.95, ISBN ??

**The Corrosion of Medicine: Can the Profession Reclaim its Moral Legacy?**
2008 / 345 pages, $24.95, ISBN ??

**Do Not Resuscitate: Why the Health Insurance Industry
is Dying, and How We Must Replace It**
2008 / 256 pages, $18.95, ISBN ??

**Hijacked: The Road to Single Payer
in the Aftermath of Stolen Healthcare Reform**
2010 / 290 pages, $18.95 / Softcover: ISBN ?? / eBook: ISBN ??

**Breaking Point: How the Primary Care Crisis
Endangers the Lives of Americans**
2011 / 234 pages, $18.95 / Softcover: ISBN 978-0-9837734-0-5
ISBN 978-0-9837734-1-2

**The Cancer Generation:
Baby Boomers Facing a perfect Storm - Second Edition**
2012 / 304 pages, $18.95 / Softcover: ISBN 978-0-9837734-3-6
eBook: ISBN 978-0-9837734-2-9

orders: www.amazon.com